Weight Wat PersonalPoints Cookbook Cookbook 2024 Edition

Taco soup recipe
Cauliflower and potato soup
Brussels sprouts & sweet potato noodle bowls
Air fryer tuna cake
Chicken stir fry recipe
Turkey taco lettuce wraps
Vegan slow cooker red lentil chili
Easy chicken corn chowder
Summer chickpea salad
Chicken tikka masala pizza
One pan balsamic chicken and veggies
Turkey avocado roll-ups
Asian chicken cranberry salad
Cauliflower and potato soup
Brussels sprouts & sweet potato noodle bowls
Air fryer tuna cake
Chicken stir fry recipe
Turkey taco lettuce wraps
Vegan slow cooker red lentil chili
Easy chicken corn chowder
Summer chickpea salad
Chicken tikka masala pizza
One pan balsamic chicken and veggies
Turkey avocado roll-ups
Asian chicken cranberry salad

Dinner Recipe

Creamy chicken and summer squash
Crockpot cranberry meatballs
Garlic brown sugar chicken
Crockpot pizza
Amish chicken corn soup
Easy slow cooker caribbean jerk chicken
Slow cooker caribbean black beans recipe
Slow cooker kalua pork with cabbage
Chicken Ranch Pasta
Weight Watchers Shredded Chicken Tacos
Thai Chicken Sheet Pan
Weight watchers crack chicken
Thai Chicken Wrap
Smothered Chicken And Gravy
Garlic brown sugar chicken
Crockpot pizza
Amish chicken corn soup
Easy slow cooker caribbean jerk chicken
Slow cooker caribbean black beans recipe
Slow Cooker Kalua Pork With Cabbage
Chicken ranch pasta
Weight watchers shredded chicken tacos
Thai Chicken Sheet Pan
Weight watchers crack chicken
Balsamic chicken

Baked buffalo chicken taquitos
Bbq chicken skewers with pineapple
Sheet pan chicken fajitas
Basil ground beef bowl
Beef enchilada casserole
One pot skillet lasagna
Roast lamb with garlic
Slow cooker pulled pork tacos
Pork tenderloin marinade
Perf

Introduction

Welcome to the all-new Weight Watchers Cookbook, your comprehensive guide to healthy, delicious, and personalized eating! In a world where wellness is a priority and balance is key, we are thrilled to present this updated cookbook tailored to your individual needs and preferences. At Weight Watchers, we understand that every person's journey to a healthier lifestyle is unique. That's why we've designed this cookbook to empower you to make food choices that align with your goals, tastes, and lifestyle.

In this latest edition, we continue our commitment to helping you achieve your weight loss and wellness goals with a fresh approach. The 2024 edition builds upon the success of our previous cookbooks, incorporating the latest nutritional science and culinary innovations to bring you a collection of mouthwatering recipes that are not only satisfying but also mindful of your PersonalPoints budget.

What Sets This Cookbook Apart?

What makes the Weight Watchers PersonalPoints Cookbook 2024 Edition truly special is its emphasis on personalization. We recognize that everyone has different dietary preferences, cultural influences, and lifestyle constraints. That's why our team of expert nutritionists and chefs have carefully crafted a diverse range of recipes that cater to various tastes and dietary requirements. Whether you're a vegetarian, a busy professional, a parent cooking for a family, or someone with specific dietary needs, you'll find recipes here that suit your lifestyle and preferences.

Highlights of the Weight Watchers PersonalPoints Cookbook 2024 Edition:

PersonalPoints System: We've revamped our Points system to make it more personalized and intuitive than ever before. Your PersonalPoints budget is calculated based on your unique profile, ensuring that you have the flexibility to enjoy your favorite foods while staying on track with your goals.

Innovative and Nutritious Recipes: Discover a wide array of recipes, from quick and easy meals for busy weekdays to elaborate dishes for special occasions. Each recipe is carefully curated to strike a balance between taste and nutrition, making your journey to a healthier you both flavorful and satisfying.

Cooking Made Easy: We understand the importance of convenience in today's fast-paced world. That's why our recipes come with easy-to-follow instructions, detailed nutritional information, and handy cooking tips, empowering you to create delicious meals with confidence.

Diverse Culinary Experience: Explore the rich tapestry of global cuisines, from Mediterranean delights and Asian-inspired dishes to classic comfort foods with a healthy twist. With our cookbook, you'll embark on a culinary adventure that tantalizes your taste buds while supporting your well-being.

Inspiration and Motivation: Beyond the kitchen, we offer motivational tips, success stories, and expert advice to keep you inspired throughout your journey. Achieving your health and wellness goals is not just about the food you eat; it's also about the mindset and support you have along the way.

We invite you to dive into the Weight Watchers PersonalPoints Cookbook 2024 Edition and embark on a transformative culinary experience. Let the flavors, textures, and aromas inspire you as you take control of your health and well-being. Get ready to savor the journey and celebrate the joy of nourishing your body and soul.

Here's to a healthier, happier you!

Warmest regards,

What Is Weight Watchers?

Weight Watchers, now known as WW International, is a popular and well-known weight loss program and commercial diet service. Founded in 1963 by Jean Nidetch, the program focuses on helping people lose weight and adopt healthier lifestyles through a combination of balanced eating, regular physical activity, and supportive community meetings.

The core concept of Weight Watchers revolves around a points system, where foods are assigned a certain number of points based on their calorie, fat, and fiber content. Members are given a daily points target and are encouraged to track their food intake to stay within their allotted points. The program promotes the consumption of nutritious foods and encourages portion control.

Over the years, Weight Watchers has evolved and introduced various iterations of its program, incorporating new research and scientific understanding of nutrition and weight management. In addition to the points system, the program emphasizes the importance of exercise, behavior modification, and emotional support in achieving long-term weight loss success.

One of the key features of Weight Watchers is its supportive community aspect. Members can attend weekly meetings, either in person or online, where they can share their experiences, receive encouragement, and get guidance from trained coaches and fellow members.

In recent years, WW International has also developed digital tools and mobile apps to help members track their progress, find recipes, and access support on the go.

How does exercise affect the WW program?

The WW program, formerly known as Weight Watchers, is a popular commercial weight loss program that emphasizes a balanced approach to nutrition and physical activity. Exercise plays a significant role in the WW program in several ways:

Activity Points: In the WW program, members are assigned a daily and weekly SmartPoints budget based on their age, weight, height, and sex. These SmartPoints are allocated for food and beverages. Exercise can help members earn additional SmartPoints, known as Activity Points, which can be used to indulge in treats or larger meals without exceeding their daily SmartPoints budget.

Promotes Overall Health: Regular exercise is essential for overall health and well-being. It can help improve cardiovascular health, increase metabolism, build muscle mass, and boost mood. Engaging in physical activity supports the WW program's holistic approach to wellness.

Boosts Weight Loss: Exercise contributes to creating a calorie deficit, which is essential for weight loss. When combined with a balanced diet and mindful eating, regular physical activity can help members achieve their weight loss goals faster and more effectively.

Increases Accountability: Participating in physical activities, whether it's going to the gym, walking, or taking fitness classes, can provide a sense of accountability. Many WW members find support and motivation by exercising with others, whether in group classes or through online communities. This accountability can help individuals stay consistent with their fitness routines.

Improves Habits: Incorporating regular exercise into one's routine can also lead to positive lifestyle changes. As members become more active, they may find themselves making healthier choices in other aspects of their lives, such as opting for nutritious meals and getting adequate sleep.

Stress Management: Exercise is known to reduce stress and anxiety levels. Managing stress is crucial for emotional well-being and can prevent emotional eating, a common challenge for many individuals trying to lose weight.

It's important to note that the impact of exercise on the WW program can vary from person to person. Some members may find that they lose weight more effectively with increased physical activity, while others might discover that exercise helps them maintain their weight loss in the long term. The key is to find enjoyable and sustainable forms of exercise that fit individual preferences and lifestyles. WW encourages its members to find activities they love, making it more likely that they will stick with their exercise routines over time.

The Function of The Smart Points System

The Smart Points system is a key component of the Weight Watchers (WW) program, which is a popular and widely used weight loss and wellness program. The system assigns a point value to every food and drink based on its nutritional content, taking into account the food's calories, saturated fat, sugar, and protein content. The main function of the Smart Points system is to help individuals make healthier food choices and manage their portion sizes while still enjoying a variety of foods.

Here's how the Smart Points system works:

1. **Point Calculation:** Each food and drink item is assigned a specific point value based on its nutritional composition. Foods high in calories, saturated fats, and sugars will have higher point values, while foods high in protein will have lower point values. This encourages members to choose foods that are lower in unhealthy fats and sugars while prioritizing lean proteins and whole foods.

2. **Personalized Daily Budget:** When individuals join the WW program, they are assigned a daily Smart Points budget based on factors like age, weight, height, and activity level. This budget represents the maximum number of points they can consume in a day while still working towards their weight loss goals.

3. **Tracking and Accountability:** Members are encouraged to track their daily food intake and stay within their Smart Points budget. This tracking can be done through the WW app or website, where they can log the foods they eat and monitor their progress. Tracking helps create awareness about eating habits and promotes accountability.

4. **Flexibility and Freedom:** The Smart Points system allows for flexibility and freedom in food choices. No foods are off-limits, but members are encouraged to make healthier choices within their daily point budget. This flexibility helps individuals learn sustainable eating habits and develop a positive relationship with food.

5. **Encourages Balanced Nutrition:** By assigning point values based on multiple nutritional factors, the system promotes a balanced and varied diet. It encourages the consumption of fruits, vegetables, lean proteins, and whole grains while discouraging excessive consumption of foods high in sugar and unhealthy fats.

6. **Supportive Community:** WW meetings and online forums provide a supportive community where members can share their experiences, struggles, and successes. This sense of community support can be instrumental in helping individuals stay motivated and committed to their weight loss journey.

Overall, the Smart Points system is designed to promote mindful eating, healthier food choices, and long-term lifestyle changes, making it easier for individuals to achieve and maintain their weight loss goals.

Advantages and disadvantages of smart points

The Smart Points System is a popular and widely used method for tracking food intake and managing weight, primarily associated with the Weight Watchers (now WW) program. This system assigns a point value to foods and beverages based on their nutritional content, encouraging individuals to make healthier food choices.

Here are the advantages and disadvantages of the Smart Points System:

Advantages:

1. **Simplicity:** The Smart Points System simplifies the process of tracking food intake. Instead of counting calories, individuals can focus on tracking points, which are assigned based on the food's nutritional value.
2. **Flexibility:** The system allows for flexibility in food choices. It encourages a balanced diet by assigning lower points to healthier foods like fruits, vegetables, and lean proteins, and higher points to less nutritious options like sugary or fatty foods. This flexibility can make it easier for individuals to adhere to the program.
3. **Encourages Healthy Choices:** By assigning lower points to healthier food options, the system promotes the consumption of nutritious foods, which can lead to better overall health.
4. **Behavioral Changes:** The Smart Points System helps individuals develop healthier eating habits by encouraging them to make mindful food choices. Over time, this can lead to long-term behavioral changes and improved overall wellness.
5. **Supportive Community:** Many people find support and motivation in the Weight Watchers community. Group meetings and online forums provide a platform for individuals to share their experiences, challenges, and successes, fostering a sense of community and accountability.

Disadvantages:

1. **Overemphasis on Points:** Some critics argue that the focus on points might lead individuals to choose low-point, processed foods over healthier, but higher-point options. This could result in a lack of important nutrients despite staying within the daily point allowance.
2. **Cost:** Participating in the official Weight Watchers program, which utilizes the Smart Points System, often requires a subscription fee. While this fee covers resources and support, it can be a financial barrier for some individuals.
3. **Potential Obsession:** For some people, constantly tracking points and food intake can lead to an unhealthy obsession with food. This can contribute to stress and anxiety, especially if individuals feel guilty about exceeding their daily point allowance.
4. **Not One-Size-Fits-All:** While the Smart Points System works well for many people, it might not be suitable for everyone. Each person's body and nutritional needs are different, and some individuals might require a more personalized approach to achieve their health and wellness goals.

5. **Limited Focus:** The Smart Points System primarily focuses on food choices and may not address other important aspects of a healthy lifestyle, such as regular physical activity and emotional well-being.

Ultimately, the effectiveness of the Smart Points System varies from person to person. Some individuals find great success and benefit from the structure and support it provides, while others may prefer different approaches to managing their weight and overall health. It's essential for individuals to find a method that works best for their unique needs and preferences.

Advantages of using weight watchers

In today's fast-paced world, where lifestyles are becoming increasingly sedentary and processed foods are readily available, obesity and related health issues have reached epidemic proportions. Individuals seeking effective and sustainable weight management solutions often find themselves overwhelmed by the multitude of diet plans and weight loss programs available in the market. Among these options, Weight Watchers stands out as a leading and time-tested program with a plethora of advantages. This article explores the numerous benefits of using Weight Watchers for achieving and maintaining a healthy weight, addressing both physical and psychological aspects of weight management.

1. Flexible and Personalized Approach

One of the key advantages of Weight Watchers is its flexibility in accommodating diverse dietary preferences and lifestyles. Unlike rigid diets, Weight Watchers employs a points-based system that assigns values to various foods based on their nutritional content. This approach allows participants to make food choices according to their preferences, making it easier to adhere to the program in the long run.

2. Scientifically Grounded Methodology

Weight Watchers' point system is backed by scientific research and nutritional expertise. The program considers factors such as calorie intake, macronutrient balance, and portion control, ensuring that participants create a calorie deficit necessary for weight loss. This evidence-based approach enhances the credibility of the program and increases the likelihood of successful outcomes.

3. Comprehensive Support System

Weight Watchers offers a robust support system through meetings, online forums, and dedicated mobile applications. Regular group meetings provide a sense of community, fostering motivation and accountability among participants. Additionally, the online platform enables individuals to track their progress, access recipes, and connect with others, creating a supportive environment conducive to achieving weight loss goals.

4. Behavioral and Psychological Support

Weight Watchers emphasizes behavioral changes and psychological support, recognizing that weight management is not merely about food choices but also about addressing emotional triggers and unhealthy habits. The program offers tools and resources to help participants develop a positive relationship with food, cope with stress, and overcome emotional eating patterns, leading to long-term success.

5. Focus on Sustainable Lifestyle Changes

Unlike quick-fix diets that often result in temporary weight loss, Weight Watchers encourages sustainable lifestyle changes. By promoting gradual and steady weight loss, the program instills healthy habits that are more likely to be maintained in the long term. Participants learn portion control, mindful eating, and regular physical activity, leading to improved overall health and well-being.

6. Incorporation of Physical Activity

Weight Watchers emphasizes the importance of regular physical activity as an integral part of a healthy lifestyle. The program encourages participants to find enjoyable forms of exercise, making it more likely for individuals to stick to their fitness routines. Physical activity not only enhances weight loss but also improves cardiovascular health, boosts metabolism, and enhances mood.

7. Professional Guidance and Expertise

Weight Watchers provides access to trained coaches and nutritionists who offer personalized guidance and support. These professionals help participants set realistic goals, modify their eating habits, and tailor the program to individual needs. The expertise of these coaches enhances the overall effectiveness of the program, ensuring that participants receive accurate information and guidance throughout their weight loss journey.

8. Long-Term Weight Maintenance

One of the most significant advantages of Weight Watchers is its focus on long-term weight maintenance. Participants are not left on their own after achieving their weight loss goals; instead, they are provided with tools and strategies to maintain their weight in the future. This ongoing support significantly reduces the chances of regaining lost weight, ensuring sustainable results.

9. Positive Impact on Health Parameters

Weight Watchers has been shown to have a positive impact on various health parameters beyond weight loss. Participants often experience improvements in blood pressure, cholesterol levels, and blood sugar levels, reducing the risk of chronic conditions such as heart disease and diabetes. These health benefits make Weight Watchers a holistic approach to overall well-being.

10. Cultivation of Healthy Eating Habits in Children

Weight Watchers offers family-friendly meal plans and encourages parents to involve their children in the process of making healthier food choices. By instilling healthy eating habits in childhood, Weight Watchers contributes to the prevention of obesity and related health issues in future generations, promoting a healthier society as a whole.

Weight Watchers offers a comprehensive and multifaceted approach to weight management that addresses the physical, psychological, and behavioral aspects of the journey. Its flexible, personalized, and scientifically grounded methodology, coupled with a robust support system and professional guidance, makes it a standout choice for individuals seeking effective and sustainable weight loss solutions. By promoting long-term lifestyle changes, encouraging physical activity, and fostering a positive relationship with food, Weight Watchers not only helps individuals achieve their weight loss goals but also improves overall health and well-being. As obesity continues to pose a significant public health challenge, Weight Watchers stands as a beacon of hope, guiding individuals toward healthier lives and brighter futures.

Banana jam recipe

Prep time: 30 minutes
Cook time: 5 minutes

Ingredients

- 2 cups of mashed bananas
- 2 cups of sugar
- 2 tbsp of lime or lemon juice

Instructions

1. Bring the water in the canner to a boil before adding the ingredients.
2. Clean the jars, bands, and tops.
3. Boiling-water sterilization makes sure the jars are free of microorganisms.
4. In a saucepan, combine all the ingredients for the banana jam and whisk often.
5. Five minutes are allotted for boiling the banana jam.
6. Spoon ladlefuls of preserves into the jars. Make sure there is at least a single inch of space above the highest thing.
7. To guarantee a tight seal, wipe the jar's rim clean with a moist cloth.
8. Please swap out the rings and caps.
9. Using the jar lifter, place the jars in the boiling water for 10 minutes.
10. Finally, remove the jars from the water bath canner using the jar lifter and place them on a towel on the counter to completely cool.

Crockpot dried fruit compote

Prep time: 10 mins
Cook time: 4 hours

Ingredients

- 5 cups of mixed dried fruits
- 2 cups of cranberry juice
- ½ cup of white zinfandel wine
- ¼ cup of fig preserves or orange marmalade
- 1 cinnamon stick, 5-inch, broken in half
- 1 tsp grated lemon zest
- 2 tsp vanilla

Instructions

1. Combine the dried fruits, cranberry juice, wine, preserves, pieces of cinnamon stick, and lemon zest in a slow cooker.
2. Cover the fruit and cook on low for 3–4 hours to soften it and thicken the sauce.
3. The slow cooker must be turned off when it is finished. Remove the sticks of cinnamon and discard them. Mix thoroughly after adding the vanilla extract.
4. Savor it, whether it's hot or cold.
5. Divide the bowl's contents among several smaller containers or into one big container. For up to four weeks, store this straightforward compote of dried fruits in the refrigerator.

Crockpot caramel recipe

Prep time: 5 minutes
Cook time: 4 hours

Ingredients

- 14 oz can of sweetened condensed milk
- 1/2 cup of butter, softened
- 1 cup of corn syrup
- 2 tsp vanilla extract
- 1 1/2 tsp lemon juice
- 1 cup of sugar
- 1 cup of brown sugar

Instructions

1. Fill your slow cooker with a casserole dish or another oven-safe container.
2. In a bowl, combine all the ingredients. Transfer to the dish for the slow cooker.
3. Fill the outside of the crock pot with warm water from the tap until the water reverses approximately two-thirds of the way up the edge of the dish. Do not yet add water to the caramel!
4. The slow cooker should be set on high for 4 to 10 hours. Please see the notes for information on how long to cook anything for to get a certain consistency.
5. Carefully remove the baking dish using oven mitts from the slow cooker. Whisk everything together quickly for about a minute, and then serve it hot.

Crockpot potatoes dijonnaise

Prep time: 15 mins
Cook time: 8 hours

Ingredients

- 1-2 tbsp dijon mustard

- 1 tbsp olive oil
- 2 tbsp red wine vinegar
- Salt and pepper as needed
- 1 tsp dried rosemary
- 4 medium potatoes, peeled and cubed
- 1 medium onion, chopped

Instructions

1. In a medium bowl, combine the mustard, oil, and vinegar. Mix everything together after adding salt and pepper. Mix to coat the potatoes and onions after adding them.
2. Spray your slow cooker with non-stick cooking spray.
3. Fill the slow cooker with the bowl's contents.
4. Cook covered on low for 8 to 10 hours, or until fork-pierced potatoes are tender.

Slow-cooker cider

Prep: 5 min.
Cook: 2 hours

Ingredients

- 2 cinnamon sticks (3 inches every)
- 1 tsp whole cloves
- 1 tsp whole allspice
- 2 quarts of apple cider
- 1/2 cup of packed brown sugar
- 1 orange, sliced

Directions

1. To create a spice bag, put the spices between two pieces of cheesecloth, collect the corners, and secure them with thread.
2. Add the cider and brown sugar to a 3-quart slow cooker and stir to combine the ingredients. Add a package of seasoning. Add orange slices on top. Cook on low heat, covered, for two to three hours, or until thoroughly heated. Throw away the spice bag.

Crock-pot easy italian beef recipe

Prep time: 10 minutes
Cook time: 8 hours

Ingredients

- 1 packet of italian beef
- 3 pounds beef pot roast

- ¾ cup of water

Instructions

1. Fill a slow cooker with at least 5 quarts with everything.
2. Cover and cook on low for 8 to 10 hours for the finest results.
3. Using two forks, shred the pot roast after removing it from the slow cooker.
4. Add the liquids and the meat back into the slow cooker.
5. Place some shredded meat on your favourite bread.

Crock-pot blueberry butter recipe

Prep time: 15 mins
Cook time: 5 hours

Ingredients

- 5 cup of blueberry
- 1 cup of granulated sugar
- 2 tsp ground cinnamon
- 1 medium lemon(zested and juiced)

Instructions

1. In the pitcher of the blender or food processor, puree or blend fresh blueberries.
2. Add the pureed blueberries, sugar, cinnamon, lemon juice, and lemon zest to a slow cooker that has a minimum 6-quart capacity if using one.
3. Cook everything on low for an hour with the lid on.
4. Support the slow cooker's cover with a wooden spoon or similar heat-safe kitchen implement to allow the liquid to evaporate.
5. For the next 4 to 5 hours, while cooking on low, check the consistency of the blueberry butter around once every hour.
6. The blueberry butter is done when it forms a nice mound on a spoon and doesn't run off.
7. Once the blueberry butter has set up, spoon it into a 1-pint jar or other food storage container and store it in the refrigerator for up to two monts or the freezer for up to a year.

Pasta primavera

Prep: 19 minutes
Cook: 11 minutes

Ingredients

- 10 oz. Dry barilla penne pasta
- Salt
- 1/4 cup of olive oil
- 1/2 medium red onion, sliced

- 1 big, peeled, and matchstick-sized carrot
- 2 cups of broccoli florets
- 1 medium red bell pepper
- 1 medium yellow squas
- 1 medium zucchini
- 3 - 4 cloves garlic cloves, minced
- 1 cup of (heaping) grape tomatoes, halved through the length
- 2 tsp dried italian seasoning
- 1/2 cup of pasta water
- 2 tbsp fresh lemon juice
- 1/2 cup of shredded parmesan
- 2 tbsp chopped fresh parsley

Instructions

1. Bring a large saucepan of water to a boil. In a saucepan of salted water, boil the penne until it is al dente. Drain, saving 1/2 cup of the cooking liquid.
2. In the meanwhile, warm the olive oil in a 12-inch (deep) skillet over medium heat.
3. After 2 minutes, add some carrot and red onion that have been chopped, and let them to simmer in the flavorful sauce that has formed.
4. Sauté the broccoli and bell pepper for 2 minutes.
5. Sauté the zucchini and squash for 2 to 3 minutes, or until they are just about ready.
6. After 2 minutes of continuous sautéing, add the garlic, tomatoes, and italian seasoning.
7. After the pasta has been drained, add the veggies, lemon juice, and more salt, if desired, to the pot or a serving dish. Toss the mixture and add some of the pasta water you set aside to thin it up if required.
8. Before serving, sprinkle with the remaining parmesan and stir in the remaining 1/4 cup of pasta.

Garlic herb baked chicken breast

Prep time: 10 mins
cook time: 20 mins

Ingredients

- 2 tbsp butter, room temperature
- 1 tsp dried parsley
- 1/2 tsp dried oregano
- 1/2 tsp dried basil
- 1/4 tsp garlic powder
- 1/4 tsp onion powder
- 1/4 tsp salt

- Freshly cracked pepper
- 2 boneless, skinless chicken breasts

Instructions

1. Increase the oven's setting to 400 degrees fahrenheit. Until the mixture resembles paste, combine the butter with the herbs and spices (parsley, oregano, basil, garlic powder, onion powder, salt, and freshly cracked pepper, if required; you'll need around 15 spins of a pepper mill).

2. Lay the chicken breasts on a cutting board, wrap them in plastic wrap, and gently pound the thick end until it is between 1/2 and 3/4 inches thick if the thickest section of the breasts is more than 3/4 inches. Dry the chicken completely with a paper towel.

3. Check that the chicken breasts on the baking sheet or in the casserole dish are separated by adequate space (a couple of inches of space between and around every breast). Apply a coating of garlic-herb butter to each breast.

4. The chicken should now be baked for 20 minutes at 400 degrees. Because chicken breasts vary in size and thickness, use a meat thermometer to check the temperature of the thickest section of the breast before taking it from the oven.

5. To ensure consistent cooking, let the chicken rest for at least five minutes after baking.

Fluffy whipped blueberry butter

Prep time: 20 minutes
Cook time: 15 minutes

Ingredients

For the blueberry sauce
- 3 cups of fresh blueberries
- 2/3 cup of sugar
- 2/3 cup of water
- 3 tablespoons of cornstarch, mixed with the same volume of cold water
- 1 tsp pure vanilla extract

For the whipped blueberry butter
- 1/4 cup of milk
- 1 cup of unsalted softened butter
- 1/3 cup of powdered sugar
- 1/3 cup of prepared blueberry sauce, cooled
- 1 tsp pure vanilla extract
- 1 pinch of kosher salt

Instructions

1. In a medium saucepan, combine the blueberries, water, and sugar. Cook, stirring occasionally, until the sugar is dissolved. Gently boil while stirring often.

2. In a cup or bowl, combine the cornstarch and water until a slurry is created. The blueberries should be incorporated very gently into the slurry. After simmering, the blueberry sauce is finished when it becomes thick enough to coat the back of a spoon. This will take 5 to 10 minutes to complete. Include the vanilla essence after turning the heat off. Until room temperature, cool. (you'll have more blueberry sauce than you'll need for the butter; it will amount to around 2-1/4 cups. Over ice cream, pancakes, and waffles, the remaining sauce is delicious.

3. A stand mixer's bowl should be used to smoothly combine milk and butter on low to medium speed. Please be patient as the ingredients may take some time to combine. The next step is to raise the speed to medium-high and beat the mixture for about 5 minutes, or until it is light and fluffy.

4. Add the salt and powdered sugar, and mix on medium-high speed for a further minute. On low speed, blend in the vanilla and a third of a cup of the blueberry sauce.

Glazed salmon with asian vegetables

Prep: 10 minutes
Cook: 15 minutes

Ingredients

- 3 x 200g skinless, boneless salmon fillets
- 1/3 cup of lee kum kee dumpling soy sauce
- 2 tbsp vegetable oil
- 1 bunch baby pak choy, trimmed
- 300g bag carrot sticks
- 200g snow peas, trimmed
- Add toasted sesame seeds and thinly sliced green spring onions as garnish.
- Steamed rice to serve

Method

1. In a large dish, combine the fish with 1 tablespoon of the sauce. Please save aside the 14 cups of sauce that are left.

2. Add half the oil to a large nonstick wok that has been preheated over high heat. Salmon should be brought in two halves. Cook until done for 4 to 5 minutes, turning once. Then proceed to a serving plate. Get warm by hiding behind anything. Wipe the wok clean.

3. In the pan, cook the remaining oil. More vegetables should be consumed. Cook veggies in a stir-fry for two minutes, or until tender. The salmon has to be returned. Stir-fry for a further minute.

4. Remove the wok from the heat. Serve the remaining sauce over top. On top, scatter some seeds and spring onions.

5. Add steamed rice as a complement.

One pan garlic herb chicken and asparagus

Prep time: 5 minutes
Cook time: 20 minutes

Ingredients

- 3-6 chicken thighs
- Salt and pepper as needed
- 1 pound asparagus - ends trimmed
- 3 tbsp butter - divided
- 1 tbsp minced garlic
- ½ tsp dried basil - (see note)
- ½ tsp dried oregano
- ½ tsp dried thyme
- ½ tsp onion powder
- Salt and pepper as needed
- Fresh herbs for garnish (optional)

Instructions

1. Be careful to season the chicken on both sides with salt and pepper. In a large skillet or pan, spread 2 tbsp of butter evenly and melt it over medium heat. Stir in the garlic and herbs after the first minute, when they are fragrant, and simmer for one more minute.
2. Chicken was placed to the pan, cooked at medium heat for the first 5-7 minutes, then turned over and cooked for an additional 5-7 minutes. (at this point, the chicken ought to have mostly finished cooking.)
3. Move the chicken to one side of the pan and fill the empty area with the remaining 1 tablespoon of butter. When the butter has melted, add the asparagus. Before serving with asparagus, season with salt and pepper as desired. Heat for 4 to 6 minutes, stirring periodically, or until veggies are tender and chicken is well cooked.
4. Add freshly cracked black pepper and, if using, fresh herbs to the serving dish right away.

3 ingredient crock pot chicken

Prep time: 1 minute
Cook time: 4 hours

Ingredients

- 2 lb boneless, skinless chicken
- 1 oz gravy packet
- 1 oz ranch packet
- 1 cup of water

Instructions

1. Lightly butter a 4-quart slow cooker and add chicken. Mix the contents of the gravy and ranch packets with the water and pour this mixture over the chicken.
2. Cook for 3-4 hour on low heat, covered.

Slow cooker beef with mushroom sauce recipe

Prep time: 15 minutes
Cook time: 6 hours

Ingredients

- 1-½ pounds lean stewing beef
- 1 medium-large onion, chopped (about 1-½ cup of)
- 2 cloves garlic, minced
- 2 cups of(8 to 10 ounces) sliced mushrooms
- 1 can (10-¾ ounces) low fat reduced sodium cream of mushroom soup
- ½ cup of dry red wine, such as merlot
- 1-½ tbsp worcester shire sauce
- 1 tsp montreal steak seasoning (optional)

Instructions

1. Add everything to the slow cooker and well combine.
2. Switch the slow cooker to the low setting, and cook the beef until it is tender, about 6 to 8 hours on low or 3.5 to 4.5 hours on high.
3. You may use cooked rice or noodles as a basis for your dish.

Weight watcher's cinnamon rolls

Prep time: 15 minutes
Cook time: 25 minutes

Ingredients

- 2 cups of self-rising flour
- 1/2 cup of + 2 tbsp powdered sugar, divided
- 1 1/2 cup of plain fat-free greek yogurt
- 1 tbsp vanilla, divided
- 1 egg
- 1 bottle of butter spray (20 sprays)
- 1/4 cup of packed brown sugar
- 1 tbsp cinnamon
- 5 sprays of cooking spray

Instructions

1. Oven temperature: 350 degrees fahrenheit.
2. Combine the flour and 2 tablespoons of powdered sugar in a large bowl. Pull back. Mix 112 cups of yogurt, 1 tablespoon of vanilla essence, and 1 egg in a medium bowl. Fold the yogurt mixture into the flour mixture and toss everything together with a wooden spoon until it is just incorporated. The dough must now be further worked with your hands in the basin until it is smooth (about 2 minutes of kneading). One tablespoon at a time, add more flour until the mixture is no longer sticky and can be worked easily.
3. Spread a large piece of parchment paper out on your desk and sprinkle some flour on it. Place the dough on the parchment paper. Roll the dough out into a 12-by-9-inch rectangle, flouring the rolling pin as necessary.
4. The dough should be thoroughly sprayed with butter spray.
5. Sprinkle cinnamon and brown sugar all the way to the borders. Roll the dough tightly, starting at one of the long ends and creating a 12-inch log with the help of parchment paper.
6. Cut the roll into 12 evenly sized pieces. The dough pieces should be arranged on an 11x7-inch baking pan that has been sprayed with cooking spray. About 22 to 25 minutes of gentle browning in the oven. Before the glaze can be applied, the food must rest for ten minutes.
7. Completely combine the yogurt, remaining 12 cups of powdered sugar, and 14 teaspoons of vanilla essence. To the cinnamon rolls, add glaze. The meal should be served hot.

Blueberry almond oatmeal

Prep: 5 min
Cook: 10 min

Ingredients

Oatmeal

- 1 cup of (81 g) rolled oats
- 2 cups of (480 ml) unsweetened almond milk†
- 1 medium banana, sliced
- ½ cup of (75 g) frozen blueberries
- 2 tbsp (14 g) ground flaxseeds
- 2 tbsp (30 ml) maple syrup
- ½ tsp pure vanilla extract
- ⅛ tsp almond extract (optional)

Toppings

- 1 medium banana, sliced
- ½ cup of (75 g) fresh blueberries
- ⅔ cup of (160 ml) unsweetened coconut yogurt‡
- 3 tbsp (45 ml) almond butter

- Optional garnish
- Ground cinnamon
- Sliced roasted almonds

Directions

1. In a saucepan, combine the oats, milk, banana, blueberries, and flaxseeds. Simmer for a few minutes. After raising to a boil, let simmer for seven minutes over low heat, stirring regularly to avoid scorching.
2. Add the maple syrup, vanilla, and almond extract after turning the burner off.
3. Spoon the porridge into bowls and top with extras like yogurt, banana slices, almond butter, and fresh fruit. Enjoy.

Strawberry smoothie

Prep time: 5 minutes
Total time: 5 minutes

Ingredients

- 1 cup of low-fat milk (or juice)
- 1/2 cup of strawberry greek yogurt
- 1 frozen banana is cut into chunks
- 1 1/2 cup of fresh or frozen strawberries

Instructions

1. Place each ingredient in the blender in the prescribed sequence.
2. Add a bit extra milk or water if the smoothie is too thick to purée. Try it out and add honey if you want it to be sweeter.

Chocolate quinoa granola bars

Prep time: 7 minutes
Cook time: 15 minutes

Ingredients

- 3.5 oz quinoa (raw)
- 1/2 cup of peanut butter
- 1/3 cup of honey
- 1/4 cup of coconut oil
- 1 & 1/3 cup of rolled oats
- 2 tbsp mixed seeds
- 2 tbsp flaked almonds
- 1 tbsp chia seeds

- 1 tbsp ground flaxseed
- 2 tbsp chocolate chips (can be dairy free)

Instructions

1. Preheat the oven to 350°f.
2. Cook the quinoa in a large pot or dish over medium heat. To achieve consistent cooking, whisk continuously for a few minutes. As the quinoa cooks, it will "pop." cook the food until the edges start to brown. Take it out of the serving dish and place it on a plate or in a different bowl.
3. Turn off the heat and whisk in the coconut oil, honey, and peanut butter to the same pot. Simmer for a few minutes until the coconut oil is melted.
4. Combine the oats, chia seeds, flaxseed, almonds—both crushed and flaked—quinoa, and chocolate chips. After vigorous mixing, the components should be well combined.
5. Place the ingredients in a parchment-lined 9 by 9-inch baking dish. Apply pressure by pressing with the back of the spoon.
6. Bake it for 15 minutes, or until the edges start to brown.
7. Before removing it from the tin and letting it cool completely, you should give it some time to cool within. And hopefully, unwind. Do this to stop further deterioration.
8. To adorn, slice the cake into 16 little bars (or 8 large bars), drizzle with melted chocolate, and then top with freeze-dried raspberries.

Vegetarian breakfast casserole
Prep:15 minutes
Cook:55 minutes

Ingredients

- 2 medium sweet potatoes peeled and diced
- 8 ounces whole cremini baby bella mushrooms
- 1 small head of broccoli cut into floret
- 1 red bell pepper diced
- 1 red or yellow onion ½-inch cut
- 1 tsp kosher salt
- ½ tsp black pepper
- 3 tbsp extra virgin olive oil
- 12 large eggs
- ½ cup of milk
- 1 garlic clove minced
- 1 ½ tsp italian seasoning herb
- 4 ounces part-skim ricotta cheese
- Chopped fresh basil

Instructions

1. Set oven racks in the top and bottom thirds and preheat to 400 degrees f. On two large baking sheets, apply a thin coating of nonstick cooking spray. Use nonstick cooking spray to coat a 9 to 13-inch baking dish, and then put it aside.
2. Place the vegetables on a large dish and drizzle with little extra virgin olive oil. Salt and pepper to taste, then combine all the ingredients. Each of the two sheets should have the vegetables spread out in a single layer. Tender vegetables will be ready in around 20 minutes if you toss the vegetables in the pan to achieve even cooking and rotate the pan placement on the upper and lower rack halfway through the roasting procedure. After that, distribute half of the roasted vegetables evenly across the casserole dish. Reduce the temperature to 350 degrees.
3. In the meanwhile, in a large mixing bowl, combine the milk, eggs, garlic, and italian spice. Transfer the mixture to the casserole with care. Place little bits of ricotta all over, then distribute the other vegetables evenly.
4. Occasionally shake the pan during baking; the casserole is finished when the center is no longer wobbly and the top is a rich golden brown color. After removing them from the oven, sprinkle fresh herbs on top. The meal should be served hot.

Keto egg muffins

Prep: 10 minutes
cook: 35 minutes

Ingredients

- 1 cup of broccoli
- 1 cup of cauliflower
- 1 cup of red bell pepper
- 2 cloves garlic
- 2 tbsp olive oil
- 8 large eggs
- 1/4 cup of heavy cream
- 1 tsp sea salt
- 1/2 tsp black pepper
- 3/4 cup of cheddar cheese

Instructions

1. As a starting point for a kitchen timer, utilize the times shown below.
2. Use a 400° fahrenheit oven to bake (204 degrees c). Line a baking sheet with foil or paper to prepare it (grease if using foil).
3. Combine the broccoli, cauliflower, red pepper, garlic powder, olive oil, and ingredients in a big bowl.

4. Arrange the vegetables on the baking sheet in an equal layer. Roasting broccoli in a warm oven for 15 to 20 minutes, or until the edges start to brown, is recommended.

5. In the meanwhile, place 12 paper or silicone liners into a muffin pan to prepare it.

6. Even after the veggies are finished cooking, the oven must remain on. Put an even layer of the veggies in the muffin tins.

7. In a dish, combine the eggs, heavy cream, sea salt, and black pepper. In the saucepan, add cheddar cheese and stir. Pour the egg mixture over the vegetables after they are placed in the muffin cups.

8. Continue baking for an additional 15 to 20 minutes, or until the eggs are set.

Hearty breakfast casserole

Prep time: 10 minutes
Cook time: 40 minutes

Ingredients

- 6 oz shredded hash browns
- 1 small red onion chopped
- 6 slices turkey bacon/bacon medallions diced
- 5 spray calorie-controlled oil
- 6 large eggs
- 1 cup of low-fat cottage cheese
- 1 cup of fat free / reduced fat shredded cheddar cheese
- ¼ tsp salt
- ¼ tsp pepper

Instructions

1. Bake at 350° fahrenheit.
Hash browns should be shredded and placed in a bowl to defrost.

3. Cut up whatever turkey bacon you use into small pieces.

4. Prepare a stovetop frying pan for medium heat by coating it with nonstick cooking spray. Add the bacon crumbles and sauté for a minute before adding the onion.

5. Sauté the bacon and onions for a further 4 to 5 minutes over medium heat, or until the bacon is browned and the onion pieces start to soften.

6. Remove it from the flames.

7. Spread the hash browns into a 9 by 6-inch casserole dish, then add the crumbled bacon and chopped onion on top.

8. Season the eggs with salt and pepper after whisking them until they have a fairly light and airy consistency.

9. The other ingredients are then topped with the cottage cheese, which has been added and blended together.

10. Add the shredded or grated cheese on top.

11. Place the dish in the middle of the oven and bake for 35 to 40 minutes, or until a knife inserted in the center comes out clean.

12. Take it out of the oven and let it cool for at least 10 minutes before slicing it into eight pieces.

13. It's up to you whether you want to eat it hot or cold!

Baked oatmeal with blueberries

Prep time: 10 minutes
Cook time: 35 minutes

Ingredients

- 1 cup of oats (80g)
- 1 medium banana
- 1 medium egg
- 1 tbsp maple syrup or honey
- 1 tsp vanilla extract
- 1 tsp cinnamon
- ½ tsp baking powder
- ⅛ tsp salt
- 1 cup of blueberries
- ½ cup of fat-free natural yogurt
- Calorie-controlled spray oil.

Instructions

1. In a separate bowl, make the banana mash.

2. Set aside separate dishes for the oats, egg, yogurt, maple syrup or honey, cinnamon, vanilla essence, and baking powder.

3. Add some mashed banana and toss to spread it throughout the mixture.

4. To get the greatest results, let the oats absorb the liquids in the mixture in the refrigerator for approximately 30 minutes. Even while it is not necessarily necessary, i believe that this additional step improves the texture of the finished product.

5. Set the oven to 350 °f.

6. Lightly spritz calorie-controlled cooking oil into a small baking dish (i used a 7-inch round baking dish).

7. Transfer half of the mixture to the dish that has been prepared and spread it out evenly after allowing it to rest for 30 minutes.

8. Top with half of the blueberries.

9. Carefully avoid squashing the berries as you sprinkle the remaining mixture on top and distribute it out to the dish's borders.

10. Next, scatter the remaining berries over the top.

11. To roast the oats, place them in the middle of the oven and cook for 30-35 minutes, or until golden brown.

12. Extra blueberries and fat-free yogurt make wonderful complements. Serve hot (or cold).

Peanut butter & banana overnight oats

Prep time: 10 minutes
Additional time: 6 hours

Ingredients

- 1 medium banana
- ½ cup of rolled oats (40g)
- ½ cup of fat-free natural yogurt
- 2 tbsp powdered peanut butter
- 1 tsp sweetener optional
- ½ tsp sugar-free chocolate syrup

Instructions

1. Cut the banana in half without peeling it. Make careful to wrap one of the pieces in plastic wrap and place it in the refrigerator for the night.
The second banana should be peeled, placed in a basin, and mashed with a fork until it is mushy.
3. Combine yogurt, milk, sugar (if using), and peanut butter with 1 tbsp of the powdered peanut butter.
4. Continue mixing everything until it is well combined.
5. After the oats have been added, stir.
6. Place in a jar, tighten the lid, and refrigerate for at least six hours.
7. Mornings are ideal for combining the leftover peanut butter powder with a little amount of water to create a thick paste.
8. Top the overnight oats with the remaining banana, peanut butter, and sugar-free chocolate syrup.

Breakfast burrito bowl with spiced butternut squash

Prep time:5 minutes
Cook time:25 minutes

Ingredients

- Cooking spray
- 20- ounces butternut squash, seeded and cut into 1-inch cubes
- 1 1/2 tsp olive oil
- 3 tsp garlic powder
- 1/2 tsp cumin

- 1/2 tsp smoked paprika
- 3/4 tsp kosher salt
- Freshly ground pepper, as needed
- 1 cup of chopped tomatoes
- 1/3 cup of chopped onion
- 1/4 cup of chopped cilantro
- Juice from ½ a lime
- Olive oil spray
- 4 large eggs
- 4 ounces hass avocado, cubed
- 1/4 cup of reduced-fat shredded cheddar cheese

Instructions

1. Preheat the oven to 425 degrees. On a large nonstick baking sheet, mist oil. In a medium bowl, combine the squash, olive oil, cumin, smoked paprika, garlic powder, 1/2 teaspoon salt, and pepper. Toss in order to coat. On a sheet pan, the squash should be equally distributed and roasted for 20 to 25 minutes, turning the pan once halfway through, or until browned and tender.
2. Prepare a small dish by combining tomatoes, onions, cilantro, lime juice, a little salt, and pepper as desired. Set aside.
3. To cook eggs to the right doneness, put them to a small pan that has been heated over medium heat, lightly mist with olive oil spray, season with salt, and cover.
4. To assemble bowls: place 1 egg, 1 ounce of avocado, 1/2 cup of pico, 1/4 cup of cheese, and 1/3 cup of squash on a plate. Continue by using the extra bowls.

Weight watchers breakfast sandwich
Prep time: 10 minutes
Cook time: 25 minutes

Ingredients

- 2 cup gold medal self rising flour
- 2 cup ofchobani greek, non-fat plain yogurt
- ½ tsp. Table salt
- ½ tsp garlic powder
- 7 large eggs
- 9 slices kroger brand fully cooked bacon
- 4.5 slices of 2% milk american cheese

Instructions

1. Increase the oven's heat to 400. As soon as there are no more crumbles, the borders of the bowl are essentially "clean," and the dough seems to be well-mixed, stop mixing the flour, salt, garlic powder, and yogurt in the bowl.
2. Spread the dough out on a surface dusted with flour. Roll out the dough to a thickness of half an inch. Use a biscuit cutter that has been sprayed with non-stick cooking spray to cut out 9 biscuits.
3. Spread non-stick cooking spray on a baking sheet and space biscuits 2 inches apart. The top should be golden brown after baking for 19 to 22 minutes.
4. While the biscuits are baking, mix 7 eggs with a fork in a medium bowl with a little salt and a dash of pepper (i use white pepper). In a large pan sprayed with nonstick cooking spray, fry eggs over low heat. Before rotating, sauté the edges until they are well done. The eggs should be cooked for a few more minutes. It should be simple to remove the cooked egg from the pan and place it on a pristine, level surface. Use your biscuit cutter to cut out nine egg circles, and then place a half-slice of cheddar on top of each one.
5. After the bacon is cooked and crispy, wipe up any lingering bacon grease with paper towels and reheat the prepared food in the microwave as directed on the box.
6. Use a knife to split the biscuit in two. An egg round with cheese and one slice of bacon are sandwiched together with the top of the biscuit.
7. After wrapping in aluminum foil, place the freezer zip bag inside. Defrosted overnight in the refrigerator, then wrapped in a paper towel and cooked for 30 to 45 seconds in the microwave.

Superfood triple berry chia pudding

Prep time:20 minutes
Cook time:0 minutes

Ingredients

- 1 cup of unsweetened almond/coconut milk beverage, used almond breeze
- 3/4 cup of fresh blueberries, blackberries, and raspberries
- 2 tbsp chia seeds
- 5-6 drops nu-naturals liquid stevia

Instructions

1. Combine the chia seeds, fruit, and almond breeze almond coconut milk in a glass container with a cover.
2. Place the jar's contents in a closed container, give it a good shake, and set it away for 15 minutes.
3. Shake it one more, then place it in the refrigerator for at least 5 to 6 hours, ideally overnight.
4. Present in two distinct bowls or glasses.

5. Enjoy!

Protein granola

Prep time: 10 minutes
Cook time: 30 minutes

Ingredients

- 1 cup of old-fashioned rolled oats
- 2 1/2 cup of crisp brown rice cereal
- 1/4 cup of unsweetened coconut flakes
- 3/4 cup of raw almonds, roughly chopped
- 3 tbsp powdered peanut butter
- 2 scoops of collagen protein powder
- 1/2 tsp kosher salt
- 1 1/2 tbsp earth balance vegan buttery sticks, melted
- 1/2 cup of unsweetened smooth applesauce
- 3 egg whites
- 2 tbsp pure maple syrup
- 1 to 2 packets of monk fruit in the raw sugar substitute or erythritol (optional)

Instructions

1. Use a 325°f oven to bake. A large baking sheet with a rim should be covered in parchment paper and placed aside.
2. In a large dish, gently combine the protein powder, salt, coconut flakes, almonds, coconut flakes, and powdered peanut butter. The vegan butter, applesauce, egg whites, and maple syrup should all be added to the center and gently folded together until combined. On the baking sheet, distribute the ingredients in an even layer.
3. To bake, place a baking sheet in the middle of an oven that has been prepared, and bake for 12 minutes. When you take it out of the oven, gently swirl it so that the ingredients are rearranged such that the center is now on the exterior and the reverse is true. Bake once more for 12 minutes in the oven. Removing the granola from the oven once more , stir in the powdered sugar substitute, if any, and serve. Re-bake for an additional 12 minutes, or until the whole thing is a rich golden brown. After taking the baking sheet out of the oven, i left the granola on it to cool and solidify. Serve immediately after cubing or breaking into tiny pieces, or store at room temperature in an airtight glass container.

Slow cooker szechuan chicken & broccoli recipe

Prep time: 15 minutes
Cook time: 3 hours

Ingredients

- 1-½ pounds boneless, skinless chicken breasts, cut into 1-inch cubes
- Salt and pepper as needed
- ½ cup of picante sauce
- 2 tbsp soy sauce
- ½ tbsp quick-cooking tapioca
- 1 cup of chopped onion
- 2 garlic cloves, minced
- ½ tsp ground ginger
- 3 cups of chopped broccoli florets
- 1 medium red pepper, cut into pieces

Instructions

1. Use nonstick cooking spray to coat the inside of your slow cooker.
2. A slow cooker should be used for the chicken.
3. Season the chicken to your tastes with salt, pepper, or any other ingredients you choose.
4. Add the other ingredients, start the slow cooker, and stir everything together.
5. To ensure the chicken is well cooked and the veggies are remain crisp-tender, cover and simmer on high for a couple of hours or on low for three or four hours, stirring often.
6. If necessary, season with more salt, pepper, and soy sauce.
7. Prepare brown rice and dish it along with more soy sauce.

Scalloped chicken and potatoes

Prep: 15 min
Total: 55 min

Ingredients

- 4.8 oz betty crocker sour cream 'n chives sliced potato mix
- 2 1/4cup of boiling water
- 3/4cup of half-and-half or whole milk
- 3cup of cubed cooked chicken
- 1cup of frozen sweet peas
- 8 oz mushroom pieces and stems, drained
- 1/2cup of progresso plain bread crumbs

- 1/4cup of butter or margarine, melted
- 1tbsp chopped fresh parsley

Instructions

1. Set oven's temperature to 450 degrees fahrenheit. In a 2-quart casserole dish, combine uncooked potato and sauce mix pouches (from the potato mix box), boiling water, half-and-half, chicken, peas, and mushrooms.
2. When the potatoes are the right level of softness, take them out of the oven and give them another spin.
3. Combine the other ingredients in a separate, small dish, and then top the potato mixture with them. Bake uncovered for a further five minutes if you want a good golden color.

Turkey sloppy joes

Prep time: 15 minutes
Cook time: 20 minutes

Ingredients

- 1 pound lean ground turkey
- 1 onion finely diced
- 2 cloves garlic minced
- 1 green bell pepper diced
- Hamburger buns and coleslaw for serving

Sauce

- 1 cup of tomato sauce
- ¼ cup of ketchup
- 1 tbsp cider vinegar
- 1 tbsp brown sugar
- 2 tsp worcestershire sauce
- 1 tsp chili powder
- 1 tsp yellow mustard

Instructions

1. In a large pan, combine the turkey, onion, and garlic. Cook over medium heat to make certain that there is no pink left. If required, the water may be emptied.
2. After the onion has turned translucent, add the green pepper and fry for a further five minutes.
3. The sauce should have thickened to your preferred consistency after cooking without the cover for around 5 to 6 minutes.
4. Distribute on hamburger buns and, if preferred, garnish with coleslaw.

Parmesan chicken meatloaf

Prep time: 20 minutes
Cook time: 1 hour

Ingredients

- 2 tbsp olive oil
- ⅓ cup of onion diced finely
- 2 cloves garlic minced
- 2 pounds of ground chicken
- ½ cup of seasoned bread crumbs
- 2 tsp milk
- ¼ cup of parmesan cheese grated
- 1 egg
- 2 tbsp fresh parsley chopped
- 1 tsp italian seasoning
- ½ tsp salt
- 3 mozzarella cheese strings cut into 1/2" slices

Topping

- ½ cup of marinara sauce
- 2 tbsp panko bread crumbs
- 1 ½ tbsp parmesan cheese grated
- 1 tbsp butter melted
- 1 tbsp fresh parsley chopped
- 1 cup of mozzarella cheese shredded

Instructions

1. Increase the oven's setting to 400 degrees fahrenheit. To line a baking sheet with foil, apply cooking spray.
2. Onions and garlic may be cooked in olive oil over a medium burner. Wait till the temperature lowers before having a meal.
3. Combine all of the meatloaf's ingredients in a big bowl and stir until everything is combined.
4. On the loaf pan, shape the mixture into an 8 by 4-inch square.
5. The dish is covered with marinara sauce and cooked for 45 minutes.
6. Combine the bread crumbs, butter, parsley, and parmesan cheese.
7. A delicious meatloaf topping is made of bread crumbs and mozzarella. Bake the loaf for a further 15-20 minutes, or until an instant-read thermometer reads 165 degrees f in the center of the loaf.
8. It is advised to wait ten minutes before cutting.

Chicken tortilla soup

prep: 10 minutes
cook: 20 minutes

Ingredients

- 1 tsp olive oil
- 1 bell pepper seeded, diced
- 1 yellow onion, diced
- 4 cloves garlic, minced
- 14.5 ounce can of diced tomatoes
- 4-ounce can of mild diced green chilies
- 5 cups of low-sodium chicken broth
- 1 tbsp chili powder
- 2 tsp ground cumin
- 1/2 tsp paprika
- 1 tsp dried oregano
- Salt and freshly ground black pepper, as need
- 15-ounce can black beans, drained and rinsed
- 2-3 boneless skinless chicken breasts
- 1 cup of frozen corn
- 1 tbsp fresh lime juice
- 1/4 cup of fresh cilantro, chopped

Instructions

1. A big saucepan should be placed over medium heat to warm the olive oil. Add the bell pepper, onion, and garlic once the onion has begun to soften, and sauté for an additional minute or so.

2. Combine some diced tomatoes, chicken broth, cumin, paprika, oregano, chili powder, and black beans. Add salt and pepper to taste. 15 to 20 minutes should be spent simmering the soup.

3. Add a few chicken pieces that have been chopped into bite-sized pieces. Continue baking the chicken for a further 7 to 10 minutes.

4. After removing the chicken from the oven, shred it with two forks. Refill the pan with the lime juice and corn.

5. Add any additional toppings you choose, such as sour cream, avocado, fresh cilantro, cheese, or shredded cheese.

Slow cooker cuban chicken with citrus recipe

Prep time: 20 mins
Cook time: 6 hrs

Ingredients

- 8 boneless skinless chicken thighs
- Salt and ground black pepper
- 1 thinly sliced yellow onion, with the skin removed.
- 8 cloves garlic, coarsely chopped
- ¾ cup of fresh orange juice
- ¾ cup of fresh lime juice
- 1 bay leaf

Instructions

1. Place the chicken in the slow cooker after generously salting and peppering it.
2. Add 1 teaspoon of salt and an equal amount of onion to the chicken.
3. Marinate the chicken in a mixture of orange, lime, and garlic juices with a bay leaf.
4. On low heat, covertly cook the chicken and onions for 6 to 8 hours. Throw the bay leaf aside after removing it. More salt and pepper should be added to the sauce as required.
5. Arrange the chicken on a plate, drizzle with some sauce, and then top with some onions.

Mel's easy slow cooker pork chops recipe
Prep time: 10 mins
Cook time: 4 hrs

Ingredients

- Nonstick spray
- 4 pork chops, about 1-inch thick (5 ounces every)
- Salt and pepper for seasoning
- 2 cloves garlic, finely minced
- ¼ cup of reduced-sodium soy sauce
- ¼ cup of low-sodium chicken broth
- 2 tbsp packed light brown sugar
- ¼ tsp red pepper flakes
- 1 tbsp instant tapioca

Instructions

1. Spray a large pan with nonstick cooking spray.
2. Be careful to season the pork chops on both sides with salt and pepper. Fry the pork chops in a skillet for 1-2 minutes on each side, or until browned.
3. A slow cooker should be filled with chops.

4. Add the garlic to the grease in the pan and stir it around until it is aromatic and browned (but not burnt; otherwise, it will turn bitter). In a bowl, whisk together the soy sauce, broth, brown sugar, and red pepper flakes. Cooking and stirring should continue while the sugar melts. Pour the tapioca over the chops after adding it to a bowl and stirring it in.

5. Put the pork chops in a covered slow cooker and simmer on low for 4 to 6 hours. Fork softness is required for the flesh.

Slow-cooker chicken pozole

Prep time: 10 mins
Total time: 6 hours 40 mins

Ingredients

- 4 c. Low-sodium chicken broth
- 3 boneless skinless chicken breasts
- 2 poblano peppers, chopped
- 1 white onion, chopped
- 2 cloves garlic, minced
- 1 tbsp. Cumin
- 1 tbsp. Oregano
- 2 tsp. Chili powder
- 2 tsp. Kosher salt
- Freshly ground black pepper
- 2 (15-oz) cans hominy, drained and rinsed
- Thinly sliced radishes, for garnish
- Sliced green cabbage for garnish
- Fresh cilantro for garnish

Directions

1. Put everything in the slow cooker except the hominy and the toppings. The chicken should be simmered on low for 6 to 8 hours, or until it is tender and cooked through, for optimal results.

2. Using two forks, remove the chicken from the slow cooker and shred it. Reintroducing the hominy to the slow cooker, it has to simmer for an additional 30 minutes.

3. Add radishes, cabbage, and cilantro to soup bowls before serving.

Crock-pot sweet acorn squash

Prep time: 10 mins
Cook time: 3 hrs

Ingredients

- 1 medium acorn squash

- 2 tbsp butter
- 2 tbsp brown sugar

Instructions

1. Remove the pulp and seeds from the acorn squashes by cutting them in half lengthwise.
2. Squash should be soft after 8 to 10 hours of slow cooking on low.
3. Use a sharp kitchen knife to carefully score the inside of the squash all over, being careful not to cut through the skin. By doing this, the butter and brown sugar will be able to penetrate the squash.
4. Divide the butter and brown sugar in half and sprinkle them equally over the squash's two halves.
5. Cook the squash, covered, on high for three hours, or until it is completely soft.
6. Serving plain or with a pinch of cinnamon and/or salt, as desired.

Easy pulled pork sandwiches

Prep: 15 mins
Cook: 9 hrs

Ingredients

- 3 tbsp brown sugar
- 3 tbsp paprika
- 1 ½ tbsp garlic powder
- 1 ½ tbsp ground black pepper
- 1 ½ tsp salt
- ½ cup of dijon mustard
- 8 pounds pork shoulder roast, rind removed
- ½ cup of barbeque sauce, or as need
- 18 large hamburger buns, split

Directions

1. The oven must be preheated to 250 degrees f before baking.
2. Combine the salt, black pepper, garlic powder, paprika, and brown sugar in a bowl to form the seasoning. Apply the full amount of the mustard and brown sugar mixture on the pork roast. A shallow baking dish should be covered with aluminum foil. A rack in a baking dish should hold a roasted pig roast.
3. Cook for 9 to 11 hours in a warm oven, or until very tender. Shred the pork into tiny pieces when it has cooled. Serve the pork on hamburger buns with some barbecue sauce mixed in to give it some moisture.

Crockpot beef and vegetable chili

Prep time: 15 mins

Cook time: 4 hrs

Ingredients

- 1 pound ground beef browned
- 3 medium zucchini peeled and chopped
- 1 medium onion chopped
- 1 green bell pepper chopped
- 1 jalapeño pepper seeded and chopped
- 1 can dice tomatoes 14.5 oz
- 1 can tomato paste. 12 oz
- 1 can kidney beans 15 oz
- 1 can black beans 15 oz
- 2 tsp minced garlic
- 1 tbsp chili powder
- 1 tsp salt
- 1 tsp cumin
- 2 cups of water

Instructions

1. Fill a slow cooker with all the ingredients. It was prepared in a 6-quart crock pot.
2. Either cooking slowly for four hours or quickly for two.

Easy italian chicken zucchini skillet
Prep: 10 mins
Cook: 19 mins

Ingredients

- 2 tbsp olive oil, divided
- 1 lb boneless, skinless chicken breasts
- 1 tsp no-salt-added italian seasoning
- 1 tsp kosher salt, divided
- 4 cups of1-inch diced zucchini
- 2 garlic cloves, finely minced or grated
- 1 15-oz can of diced tomatoes
- 1 tbsp tomato paste
- 1/2 cup of chicken stock
- 2 tbsp butter
- 1/4 cup of lightly packed fresh basil, thinly sliced
- Red pepper flakes as needed

Instructions

1. In a 12-inch deep pan over medium heat, warm 1 tablespoon of olive oil. The chicken should be mixed in, with the pieces being careful not to touch or overlap. Stir in the italian spice and half a teaspoon of salt.
2. If you cook the chicken for approximately 5 minutes without rotating it, the outside may get golden brown. Cook for a further 3 minutes, turning just once, or until slightly cooked through and browned on both sides. Remove from the frying and set aside.
3. In the same skillet, warm the additional tablespoon of olive oil over low heat. Include the zucchini, add the salt and pepper, and boil for 5 minutes while stirring often.
4. Add the garlic and cook, stirring often, for about a minute, or until the scent comes out.
5. Add the tomato paste and chopped tomatoes to the pan after adding the chicken stock and stirring.
6. After the chicken has finished cooking, add it back to the pan, reduce the heat to medium-low, and simmer it covered for 5 minutes.
7. After taking the pan from the heat, add the butter and stir to combine. Take a taste of the sauce and, if necessary, season it with extra salt. Serving with a sprinkle of fresh basil and red pepper flakes.

Slow cooker chicken, broccoli, and rice casserole
prep time: 10 mins
cook time : 3 hrs

Ingredients

- 1 small onion (chopped)
- 1 cup of long grain brown rice
- 1 tbsp dijon mustard
- 1 tsp garlic powder
- 1 tsp dried thyme
- 1/2 tsp salt
- 1/4 tsp black pepper
- 2 cup low sodium chicken broth
- 1 pound boneless skinless chicken breasts
- 1 pound broccoli (cut into small pieces)
- 1/2 cup of plain greek yogurt (optional for extra creaminess)
- 1/2 cup of grated parmesan cheese
- 1 cup of shredded cheddar cheese

Instructions

1. Arrange onion, brown rice, dijon mustard, garlic powder, dried thyme, salt, and pepper in a layer at the bottom of a slow cooker.

2. After adding it and thoroughly combining it, incorporate the broth.

3. Chicken is required for the crock pot. To the chicken, add a bit extra freshly ground black pepper.

4. Cook on high heat, covered, for 2 1/2 to 3 1/2 hours, or until the chicken is well cooked and the rice has soaked up nearly all of the liquid. This took my slow cooker three hours on high to finish.

5. After the slow cooking phase, prepare the broccoli. It may be microwaved, roasted in a regular oven, or steam-cooked in a pot. (broccoli may also be prepared in a slow cooker by adding it on top of the chicken and rice during the last hour of cooking. If cooked slowly, broccoli loses its vibrant green color. I've found that boiling the broccoli in a saucepan on the stove yields the best results.

6. When the rice has finished cooking, remove the chicken from it and place it on a cutting board.

7. Combine the rice in the slow cooker with the plain greek yogurt, parmesan cheese, and cheddar cheese. Stir it well to combine the flavors.

8. Cut the chicken into pieces and add it to the cooked broccoli in the slow cooker. Mix thoroughly after adding .

Taco soup recipe

Prep: 10 minutes
Cook: 35 minutes

Ingredients

- 2 tsp olive oil
- 1 1/4 lbs lean ground beef
- 1 1/2 cup yellow onion chopped
- 2 cloves garlic, minced
- 1 jalapeno, seeded and finely chopped
- 2 (14.5 oz) cans diced tomatoes with green chiles
- 1 (14 oz) can of low-sodium beef broth
- 1 (8 oz) can tomato sauce
- 1 tbsp chili powder
- 1 tsp ground cumin
- 3/4 tsp ground paprika
- 1/4 tsp dried oregano
- 1 1/2 tbsp dry ranch dressing mix
- Salt and freshly ground black pepper
- 1 1/2 cup of frozen corn
- 14.5 oz black beans, drained and rinsed
- 14.5 oz pinto beans, drained and rinsed

Instructions

1. Heat the oil in a large saucepan over medium heat.
2. In the large pan, combine the chopped onion and crumbled ground meat. Add the jalapeño and garlic when the onion has become translucent, and sauté for an additional minute.
3. Trim off all the excess fat if you're using ground beef.
4. Add the tomato-chile combination, beef broth, tomato sauce, chili powder, cumin, paprika, oregano, ranch dressing mix, and any other spices you choose after seasoning with salt and pepper as necessary. With the lid on, simmer for 30 minutes while monitoring and stirring often.
5. Continue cooking until the pinto, black, and corn beans are heated. Add a half cup of water to the soup to change the consistency. If you have lime and cilantro, use them.
6. After adding your preferred toppings, serve the hot meal.

Cauliflower and potato soup
Prep time: 15 minutes
Cook time: 25 minutes

Ingredients

For the soup:
- 2 tbsp extra virgin olive oil
- 1 large brown/yellow onion – roughly chopped
- 3 cloves garlic – peeled and chopped
- 17 ounces cauliflower – divided into florets
- 2 medium potatoes – peeled and chopped
- 3 cup of vegetable stock
- 2 tsp fresh thyme leaves
- Sea salt and black pepper as needed
- ¼ cup of fresh parsley leaves

To garnish: (optional)
- Fresh parsley leaves
- Finely grated lemon zest

Instructions

1. A large saucepan should be used to heat the olive oil over medium heat.
2. After sautéing the onion for about 5 minutes, avoid letting it brown.
3. After placing it in the pan, sauté the garlic for around two minutes. Take care to prevent it from catching fire.
4. Add the potatoes, vegetable stock, cauliflower florets, and thyme leaves.
5. When necessary, add salt and freshly ground pepper.
6. After cooking the mixture at a low boil for 15 minutes, the vegetables need to be tender.

7. After you turn off the heat and swirl the pan, you should add the parsley.

8. To create a silky purée, you may use a blender or a hand mixer.

9. Reheat to a simmer in a pot, adding salt and pepper as required.

10. Add freshly cut parsley and thinly sliced lemon peel to each dish as a garnish.

Brussels sprouts & sweet potato noodle bowls

Prep time: 15 minutes

Cook time: 20 minutes

Ingredients

- 2 medium sweet potatoes
- 1 tsp curry powder
- ¾ pound brussels sprouts
- 4 strips center cut bacon
- 1/3 heaping cup of pecans
- ½ small red onion
- 1 tbs fresh thyme leaves
- Black pepper and kosher salt, if required

Vinaigrette:

- 1 tbs apple cider vinegar
- 1 tbs grainy dijon mustard
- 2 tbs pure maple syrup
- 1 clove garlic - peeled
- 1/3 cup of canola oil

Instructions

1. To fry bacon to the desired crispness, sauté it in a large skillet over medium heat for approximately 7 minutes. Transfer the bacon to a dish covered in paper towels with a slotted spoon so it can drain. Place all of the bacon fat—all except one tablespoon—in a bowl (you will use this later)

2. Make the topping in the interim: place everything in the bowl of a small food processor and pulse until smooth (oil not included). Process everything in a blender. While the processor is running, oil should be slowly added. Continue processing the combination until it is thoroughly emulsified and smooth. Salt & pepper to taste. Put into a mason jar with a tight-fitting cover. Unless necessary, stay out of the way.

3. Before adding the sweet potato noodles, season the pan with salt, pepper, and curry powder. Cook for 5-8 minutes, stirring occasionally, or until noodles are cooked but still firm. To keep the noodles warm, cram them into a large bowl and cover with foil.

4. Add the tbsp of bacon grease you previously left aside and bring the pan (or oil) back to medium heat. Add some brussels sprouts and onions. The dish requires pepper and salt. Wait 4 to 5 minutes, stirring often, until the sprouts start to brown. Add the pecans and thyme. Cooking the sprouts for one more minute will gently sear the sprouts and toast the nuts.

5. Top the dish of sweet potato noodles with sprouts. Make sure the bacon is evenly divided before adding it. Vinaigrette may be re-emulsified by aggressively shaking it. Stir the salad while adding the first half of the dressing.

6. To serve, divide the noodles among dishes. Fresh thyme sprigs may be used as a garnish along with more vinaigrette on the side.

Air fryer tuna cake

Ingredients

- 2 - 12 oz. Cans of chunk tuna in water
- 2 eggs
- 1/2 cup of seasoned breadcrumbs
- 4 tbsp. Mayo
- 2 tbsp. Lemon juice
- 1/2 diced white onion
- 1/2 tsp. Salt
- 1/2 tsp. Black pepper

Instructions

1. Strain the tuna and then place it in a large basin. Add the other ingredients and combine them carefully with your hands. Keep in mind that the combination should be rather stiff. Add a few more breadcrumbs to make it less mushy.

2. The air fryer basket may be greased with cooking spray or olive oil.

3. Form the ingredients into four or so patties, then place them in the air fryer's basket. If you need to flip them, leave some room between them.

4. Prepare for 12 minutes with a single flip in a 375°f oven. Repeat until all of the patties are finished, then remove and set aside. The food has to be served immediately.

Chicken stir fry recipe

Prep time: 5 minutes
Cook time: 15 minutes

Ingredients

- 1 lb of chicken breast, cut into stir-fry strips
- 2 large carrots
- 1 head broccoli
- 1 red bell pepper
- 1-2 cups of fresh spinach

For the sauce:
- 1/2 cup of soy sauce
- 1 tsp sesame oil
- 1/2 tsp ground ginger
- 1 tsp sugar
- 2 tsp cornstarch

Instructions

1. To create the sauce, mix the soy sauce, sesame oil, ginger, sugar, and cornstarch in a small basin. The tastes should be well mixed together. As an alternative, i'll prepare the sauce in advance by mixing the ingredients in a jar, keeping it in the refrigerator, and shaking it vigorously before adding it to the pan.

2. Ensure that the vegetables are tidy and cut into manageable pieces. Matchstick-sized carrots, tiny broccoli blossoms, and long strips of bell pepper were among my preparations.

3. Heat a sizable skillet or wok on medium-high with a thin layer of oil. The chicken should cook for three to four minutes, or until the outside is no longer pink, after being added.

4. Add some pepper, carrots, and broccoli to the pan. Stir. Cook the vegetables for 5-7 minutes, or until they start to soften.

5. Combine some sauce and spinach in a skillet. Reduce the temperature to low-medium. Stir after around 5 minutes in the pan, the spinach should have wilted and the sauce should have thickened.

6. Turn off the heat and stir in the lemon juice, if using. Serve your rice with a sprinkle of sesame seeds.

Turkey taco lettuce wraps

Prep: 5 minutes
Cook: 12 minutes

Ingredients

- 1 tbsp olive oil
- 3/4 cup of chopped yellow onion
- 1 lb 95% lean ground turkey
- 2 cloves garlic
- Salt and freshly ground black pepper
- 1 tbsp chili powder
- 1 tsp ground cumin
- 1/2 tsp paprika
- 1/2 cup of tomato sauce
- 1/2 cup of low-sodium chicken broth
- Iceberg or romain lettuce leaves

Instructions

1. A nonstick pan should be prepared with olive oil over medium heat.
2. Add the onion and sauté until transparent for the following two minutes. After adding the turkey, sauté the garlic for approximately 5 minutes, breaking up and stirring the meat occasionally.
3. Add salt, pepper, cumin, paprika, tomato paste, chili powder, and chicken stock for seasoning. For approximately 5 minutes, or when the sauce has reduced, keep at a low boil.
4. Place the mixture into lettuce leaves and then top.

Vegan slow cooker red lentil chili

Prep time: 10 mins
Cook time: 3 hours

Ingredients

- 1 medium white or yellow onion, diced
- 2 bell peppers
- 1 carrot, peeled and diced
- 1 jalapeño, deseeded and minced
- 3 cloves garlic, minced
- 2 tbsp chili powder
- 2 tsp ground cumin
- 1 tsp dried oregano
- 1 tsp regular or smoked paprika
- 1 28 oz. Can diced tomatoes with the juices
- 2 tbsp tomato paste
- 3–4 cups of vegetable broth
- 2 cups of dry red lentils
- Sea salt and black pepper, as need

Instructions

1. Everything has to be combined and put in a slow cooker.
2. Cook on high for 3 hours or in the slow cooker for 5 to 6 hours.
3. Next, top with your chosen chili toppings, including salsa, chopped scallions, vegan sour cream, avocado, and dairy-free cheese. Then, serve right immediately.

Easy chicken corn chowder

Prep time: 25 mins
Cook time: 15 mins

Ingredients

- 1 tbsp butter
- 1/2 cup of finely chopped onion
- 1/2 cup of finely chopped celery
- 1 medium jalapeno pepper, seeded and minced
- 2 tbsp all-purpose flour
- 3 cups of 2% milk
- 2 cups of chopped roasted, skinless, boneless chicken breasts
- One 14.75-ounce can cream style corn
- 1½ cup of frozen corn kernels (or 3 ears of fresh corn)
- 1½ tsp chopped fresh thyme
- 1/2 tsp salt
- 1/8 tsp ground red pepper

Instructions

1. In a large saucepan, melt the butter over low to medium heat. Add the onion, celery, and jalapeño after 2 minutes, then simmer for a further 3 minutes, stirring regularly, or until the vegetables are soft.
2. After adding the flour, boil the mixture for a minute while stirring constantly. Mixing the milk with the other ingredients is necessary.
3. Raise the heat and let it boil until it thickens (about 5 minutes.)

Summer chickpea salad
Prep time: 20 minutes
Total time: 20 minutes

Ingredients

- 15-ounce can chickpeas, rinsed and drained
- 1 1/2 cup of chopped persian cucumbers
- 1 cup of cherry tomatoes, halved
- 1 cup of fresh or frozen (defrosted) corn
- 1 pevery, diced
- 1 jalapeño, seeded and minced
- 1 tbsp finely chopped chives
- 1/4 cup of basil leaves, chopped
- 1/2 cup of cubed or crumbled feta cheese
- 1/4 cup of fresh lemon juice
- 1 1/2 tbsp olive oil
- 1 tbsp dijon mustard

- 1 tbsp honey
- Black pepper, freshly ground, and kosher salt as desired

Instructions

1. Combine the chickpeas, feta, tomatoes, cucumbers, peas, corn, jalapenos, basil, and chives in a large bowl.
2. In a small bowl, combine the lemon juice, dijon mustard, honey, olive oil, salt, and pepper. Mix the salad well with the vinaigrette after adding it. When you're ready to eat, taste the food for seasoning and either serve right away or cover and refrigerate.

Chicken tikka masala pizza

Prep time20 minutes
Cook time15 minutes

Ingredients

- 10 oz. Skinless and boneless chicken breast
- 1 tbsp butter
- 2 cloves garlic, minced
- 1/2 jalapeno, deseeded

Salt as need

- 1 12-inches store-bought pizza crust
- Olive oil for brushing
- 1/4 onion, thinly sliced
- 1 cup of mozzarella cheese
- A handful of coriander leaves

Marinade:

- 1/2 tsp ground cumin
- 1/2 tsp ground cayenne pepper
- 1/2 tsp ground garam masala
- 1/2 tsp minced fresh ginger
- 1/4 tsp salt
- 1/4 tsp ground black pepper
- 1 tbsp lemon juice
- 2 tbsp plain yogurt
- 1 pinch cinnamon

Tomato sauce:

- 4 oz. (115 g) tomato sauce
- 2 tbsp plain yogurt
- 2 tbsp heavy cream

Spice mix:

- 1/2 tsp cumin
- 1/2 tsp paprika
- 1/2 tsp garam masala

Instructions

1. Put the chicken and marinade in a bowl, and let them both marinate for at least an hour.

2. Line a grilling pan with aluminum foil to prepare it. After removing the chicken from the marinade, arrange it in a single layer on the pan. During the 6-7 minute grilling session at 450 degrees fahrenheit, flip the chicken halfway (232 degrees celsius).

3. While the chicken cooks, place bowls of tomato sauce and spice mix on the table. When the chicken is finished, remove it from the pan and discard the cooking liquid.

4. In a small saucepan over low heat, melt the butter. Jalapeno and garlic need to be sautéed until fragrant. When the stew starts to smell good, add the spice mix and simmer for a further 1-2 minutes, stirring periodically. Once the jalapeño has been taken out, throw it away.

5. Add the tomato sauce and thoroughly combine. Salt to taste, then boil for an additional two minutes to thicken the sauce. Remove the chicken from the fire and mix it into the sauce after it has finished cooking.

6. Before using the oven, it is advised that it be heated to 450 degrees fahrenheit (232 degrees celsius). Pizza dough should be placed on a pizza pan that has been lightly greased with olive oil. Sauce or gravy should be applied to the pizza dough. Add a quarter cup of cheese on top. Place the chicken and pizza together. Add some chopped cilantro, thinly sliced onions, and any remaining cheese to finish it off.

7. Lower the oven's temperature to 425 degrees fahrenheit (218 degrees celsius). Bake the pizza for 8 to 10 minutes on the oven's timer. Take the pizza out of the oven once it has finished cooking, then top it with the remaining cilantro that has been chopped.

One pan balsamic chicken and veggies

Prep time: 10 minutes
Cook time: 20 minutes

Ingredients

- 6 tbsp balsamic vinegar
- 1/2 cup of zesty italian dressing
- 1.25 pounds of chicken tenders
- 2 heads broccoli
- 1 cup of baby carrots
- 1/2 pint cherry tomatoes
- 1 tsp italian seasoning
- 3 tbsp olive oil
- 1/2 tsp garlic powder

- Optional: fresh parsley, salt, and pepper

Instructions

1. Preheat the oven to 400°f. Prepare a large baking sheet by spraying it with nonstick spray (or coating it with parchment paper if your tray isn't already nonstick) to avoid the balsamic and italian spice mixture from sticking.
2. Combine the spicy italian dressing and balsamic vinegar in a blender.
3. Trim the tenderloins of any excess fat and gristle. Alternately, cut the breasts into quarter- to half-inch-thick, bite-sized chunks.
4. Place the chicken tenders in a big plastic bag along with 1/3 cup of the italian spice and balsamic vinegar mixture, and shake vigorously. Marinate for a minimum of 30 minutes and a maximum of 6 hours, coating and chilling in between.
5. Separate the broccoli into bite-sized pieces. Cut the little carrots in half lengthwise.
6. Arrange broccoli, carrots, and cherry tomatoes on the baking sheet that has been prepped (would you want your tomatoes to be less roasted? After the broccoli and carrots have cooked for 5 to 10 minutes, toss in. They are already pretty soft, unless specifically specified differently.) Garlic powder, olive oil, italian seasoning, and more salt and pepper to taste.
7. The veggies just need to cook for ten to fifteen minutes.
8. Remove it from the oven, then turn it over. As seen in the video, arrange the veggies on the tray's two sides, followed by the chicken tenders (just touched by marinade). Use 1/3 cup of the balsamic and italian concoction to coat the chicken.
9. Depending on the size of your chicken, put back in the oven and cook for a further 7 to 15 minutes. You must keep a close eye on the chicken to prevent overcooking. The size of the chicken has a big impact on how long it takes to cook.
10. The remaining chicken and veggies may be served with the balsamic and italian sauce. Before serving, those who would like might garnish with freshly chopped parsley.
11. Excellent with quinoa or rice as a grain.

Turkey avocado roll-ups
prep time: 10 minutes
cook time :1 minute

Ingredients

- 2 large tortillas or wraps
- 1/2 cup of simply avocado dip and spread your choice of flavor
- 1/2 lb thinly sliced smoked turkey
- 1 1/4 cup of spinach leaves
- 4 slices of swiss cheese
- 3 slices bacon

Instructions

1. Lay out the tortillas. Each tortilla should include a quarter cup of simply avocado.
2. Place the turkey, spinach, swiss cheese, and bacon on one-third of the tortilla after spreading half of the avocado on it.
3. After gathering your garnishes, roll the tortilla starting at the end.
4. To serve, slice the dish into pinwheels.

Asian chicken cranberry salad

Prep time: 15 mins
Total time: 15 mins

Ingredients

- 2 small bags of coleslaw mix
- 4 cups of rotisserie chicken, finely chopped
- 1 ½ cup of toasted sliced almonds,
- 1 ½ cup of dried cranberries
- ¾ cup of red onion, finely diced
- 1 cup of sesame sticks
- 1 ½ cup of chopped cilantro
- 1-2 small cans of mandarin oranges, drained
- ¼ cup of black sesame seeds
- 1 cup of extra-virgin olive oil
- ½ cup of balsamic vinegar
- 4 tbsp. Low-sodium soy sauce
- 3-4 cloves garlic, chopped
- 4 tbsp. Honey or brown sugar
- 4 tbsp. Minced ginger
- 2 tsp. Toasted sesame oil

Instructions

1. A large dish is piled with cabbage, chicken, almonds, cashews, cranberries, red onion, sesame seeds, sesame sticks (optional), and fresh cilantro. Mandarin oranges need to be included (optional).
2. Combine the sesame oil, garlic, honey, balsamic vinegar, olive oil, and ginger in a blender. Add 3 tablespoons of water. Blend until completely smooth.
3. Drizzle the dressing sparingly over the ingredients for a more or less sloppy salad. After a quick toss, serve.

Cauliflower and potato soup

Prep time: 15 minutes

Cook time: 25 minutes

Ingredients

For the soup:

- 2 tbsp extra virgin olive oil
- 1 large brown/yellow onion – roughly chopped
- 3 cloves garlic – peeled and chopped
- 17 ounces cauliflower – divided into florets
- 2 medium potatoes – peeled and chopped
- 3 cup ofvegetable stock
- 2 tsp fresh thyme leaves
- Sea salt and black pepper as needed
- ¼ cup of fresh parsley leaves

To garnish: (optional)

- Fresh parsley leaves
- Finely grated lemon zest

Instructions

1. A large saucepan should be used to heat the olive oil over medium heat.
2. After sautéing the onion for about 5 minutes, avoid letting it brown.
3. After placing it in the pan, sauté the garlic for around two minutes. Take care to prevent it from catching fire.
4. Add the potatoes, vegetable stock, cauliflower florets, and thyme leaves.
5. When necessary, add salt and freshly ground pepper.
6. After cooking the mixture at a low boil for 15 minutes, the vegetables need to be tender.
7. After you turn off the heat and swirl the pan, you should add the parsley.
8. To create a silky purée, you may use a blender or a hand mixer.
9. Reheat to a simmer in a pot, adding salt and pepper as required.
10. Add freshly cut parsley and thinly sliced lemon peel to each dish as a garnish.

Brussels sprouts & sweet potato noodle bowls

Prep time: 15 minutes
Cook time: 20 minutes

Ingredients

- 2 medium sweet potatoes
- 1 tsp curry powder
- ¾ pound brussels sprouts
- 4 strips center cut bacon
- 1/3 heaping cup of pecans

- ½ small red onion
- 1 tbs fresh thyme leaves
- Black pepper and kosher salt, if required

Vinaigrette:
- 1 tbs apple cider vinegar
- 1 tbs grainy dijon mustard
- 2 tbs pure maple syrup
- 1 clove garlic - peeled
- 1/3 cup of canola oil

Instructions

1. To fry bacon to the desired crispness, sauté it in a large skillet over medium heat for approximately 7 minutes. Transfer the bacon to a dish covered in paper towels with a slotted spoon so it can drain. Place all of the bacon fat—all except one tablespoon—in a bowl (you will use this later)

2. Make the topping in the interim: place everything in the bowl of a small food processor and pulse until smooth (oil not included). Process everything in a blender. While the processor is running, oil should be slowly added. Continue processing the combination until it is thoroughly emulsified and smooth. Salt & pepper to taste. Put into a mason jar with a tight-fitting cover. Unless necessary, stay out of the way.

3. Before adding the sweet potato noodles, season the pan with salt, pepper, and curry powder. Cook for 5-8 minutes, stirring occasionally, or until noodles are cooked but still firm. To keep the noodles warm, cram them into a large bowl and cover with foil.

4. Add the tbsp of bacon grease you previously left aside and bring the pan (or oil) back to medium heat. Add some brussels sprouts and onions. The dish requires pepper and salt. Wait 4 to 5 minutes, stirring often, until the sprouts start to brown. Add the pecans and thyme. Cooking the sprouts for one more minute will gently sear the sprouts and toast the nuts.

5. Top the dish of sweet potato noodles with sprouts. Make sure the bacon is evenly divided before adding it. Vinaigrette may be re-emulsified by aggressively shaking it. Stir the salad while adding the first half of the dressing.

6. To serve, divide the noodles among dishes. Fresh thyme sprigs may be used as a garnish along with more vinaigrette on the side.

Air fryer tuna cake
Ingredients
- 2 - 12 oz. Cans of chunk tuna in water
- 2 eggs
- 1/2 cup of seasoned breadcrumbs
- 4 tbsp. Mayo
- 2 tbsp. Lemon juice
- 1/2 diced white onion

- 1/2 tsp. Salt
- 1/2 tsp. Black pepper

Instructions

1. Strain the tuna and then place it in a large basin. Add the other ingredients and combine them carefully with your hands. Keep in mind that the combination should be rather stiff. Add a few more breadcrumbs to make it less mushy.
2. The air fryer basket may be greased with cooking spray or olive oil.
3. Form the ingredients into four or so patties, then place them in the air fryer's basket. If you need to flip them, leave some room between them.
4. Prepare for 12 minutes with a single flip in a 375°f oven. Repeat until all of the patties are finished, then remove and set aside. The food has to be served immediately.

Chicken stir fry recipe

Prep time: 5 minutes
Cook time: 15 minutes

Ingredients

- 1 lb of chicken breast, cut into stir-fry strips
- 2 large carrots
- 1 head broccoli
- 1 red bell pepper
- 1-2 cups of fresh spinach

For the sauce:
- 1/2 cup of soy sauce
- 1 tsp sesame oil
- 1/2 tsp ground ginger
- 1 tsp sugar
- 2 tsp cornstarch

Instructions

1. To create the sauce, mix the soy sauce, sesame oil, ginger, sugar, and cornstarch in a small basin. The tastes should be well mixed together. As an alternative, i'll prepare the sauce in advance by mixing the ingredients in a jar, keeping it in the refrigerator, and shaking it vigorously before adding it to the pan.
2. Ensure that the vegetables are tidy and cut into manageable pieces. Matchstick-sized carrots, tiny broccoli blossoms, and long strips of bell pepper were among my preparations.
3. Heat a sizable skillet or wok on medium-high with a thin layer of oil. The chicken should cook for three to four minutes, or until the outside is no longer pink, after being added.
4. Add some pepper, carrots, and broccoli to the pan. Stir. Cook the vegetables for 5-7 minutes, or until they start to soften.

5. Combine some sauce and spinach in a skillet. Reduce the temperature to low-medium. Stir after around 5 minutes in the pan, the spinach should have wilted and the sauce should have thickened.

6. Turn off the heat and stir in the lemon juice, if using. Serve your rice with a sprinkle of sesame seeds.

Turkey taco lettuce wraps

Prep: 5 minutes
Cook: 12 minutes

Ingredients

- 1 tbsp olive oil
- 3/4 cup of chopped yellow onion
- 1 lb 95% lean ground turkey
- 2 cloves garlic
- Salt and freshly ground black pepper
- 1 tbsp chili powder
- 1 tsp ground cumin
- 1/2 tsp paprika
- 1/2 cup of tomato sauce
- 1/2 cup of low-sodium chicken broth
- Iceberg or romain lettuce leaves

Instructions

1. A nonstick pan should be prepared with olive oil over medium heat.

2. Add the onion and sauté until transparent for the following two minutes. After adding the turkey, sauté the garlic for approximately 5 minutes, breaking up and stirring the meat occasionally.

3. Add salt, pepper, cumin, paprika, tomato paste, chili powder, and chicken stock for seasoning. For approximately 5 minutes, or when the sauce has reduced, keep at a low boil.

4. Place the mixture into lettuce leaves and then top.

Vegan slow cooker red lentil chili

Prep time: 10 mins
Cook time: 3 hours

Ingredients

- 1 medium white or yellow onion, diced
- 2 bell peppers
- 1 carrot, peeled and diced
- 1 jalapeño, deseeded and minced

- 3 cloves garlic, minced
- 2 tbsp chili powder
- 2 tsp ground cumin
- 1 tsp dried oregano
- 1 tsp regular or smoked paprika
- 1 28 oz. Can diced tomatoes with the juices
- 2 tbsp tomato paste
- 3–4 cups of vegetable broth
- 2 cups of dry red lentils
- Sea salt and black pepper, as need

Instructions

1. Everything has to be combined and put in a slow cooker.
2. Cook on high for 3 hours or in the slow cooker for 5 to 6 hours.
3. Next, top with your chosen chili toppings, including salsa, chopped scallions, vegan sour cream, avocado, and dairy-free cheese. Then, serve right immediately.

Easy chicken corn chowder
Prep time: 25 mins
Cook time: 15 mins

Ingredients

- 1 tbsp butter
- 1/2 cup of finely chopped onion
- 1/2 cup of finely chopped celery
- 1 medium jalapeno pepper, seeded and minced
- 2 tbsp all-purpose flour
- 3 cups of 2% milk
- 2 cups of chopped roasted, skinless, boneless chicken breasts
- One 14.75-ounce can cream style corn
- 1½ cup of frozen corn kernels (or 3 ears of fresh corn)
- 1½ tsp chopped fresh thyme
- 1/2 tsp salt
- 1/8 tsp ground red pepper

Instructions

1. In a large saucepan, melt the butter over low to medium heat. Add the onion, celery, and jalapeño after 2 minutes, then simmer for a further 3 minutes, stirring regularly, or until the vegetables are soft.

2. After adding the flour, boil the mixture for a minute while stirring constantly. Mixing the milk with the other ingredients is necessary.

3. Raise the heat and let it boil until it thickens (about 5 minutes.)

Summer chickpea salad

Prep time: 20 minutes
Total time: 20 minutes

Ingredients

- 15-ounce can chickpeas, rinsed and drained
- 1 1/2 cup of chopped persian cucumbers
- 1 cup of cherry tomatoes, halved
- 1 cup of fresh or frozen (defrosted) corn
- 1 pevery, diced
- 1 jalapeño, seeded and minced
- 1 tbsp finely chopped chives
- 1/4 cup of basil leaves, chopped
- 1/2 cup of cubed or crumbled feta cheese
- 1/4 cup of fresh lemon juice
- 1 1/2 tbsp olive oil
- 1 tbsp dijon mustard
- 1 tbsp honey
- Black pepper, freshly ground, and kosher salt as desired

Instructions

1. Combine the chickpeas, feta, tomatoes, cucumbers, peas, corn, jalapenos, basil, and chives in a large bowl.

2. In a small bowl, combine the lemon juice, dijon mustard, honey, olive oil, salt, and pepper. Mix the salad well with the vinaigrette after adding it. When you're ready to eat, taste the food for seasoning and either serve right away or cover and refrigerate.

Chicken tikka masala pizza

Prep time20 minutes
Cook time15 minutes

Ingredients

- 10 oz. Skinless and boneless chicken breast
- 1 tbsp butter
- 2 cloves garlic, minced
- 1/2 jalapeno, deseeded

Salt as need
- 1 12-inches store-bought pizza crust
- Olive oil for brushing
- 1/4 onion, thinly sliced
- 1 cup of mozzarella cheese
- A handful of coriander leaves

Marinade:
- 1/2 tsp ground cumin
- 1/2 tsp ground cayenne pepper
- 1/2 tsp ground garam masala
- 1/2 tsp minced fresh ginger
- 1/4 tsp salt
- 1/4 tsp ground black pepper
- 1 tbsp lemon juice
- 2 tbsp plain yogurt
- 1 pinch cinnamon

Tomato sauce:
- 4 oz. (115 g) tomato sauce
- 2 tbsp plain yogurt
- 2 tbsp heavy cream

Spice mix:
- 1/2 tsp cumin
- 1/2 tsp paprika
- 1/2 tsp garam masala

Instructions

1. Put the chicken and marinade in a bowl, and let them both marinate for at least an hour.
2. Line a grilling pan with aluminum foil to prepare it. After removing the chicken from the marinade, arrange it in a single layer on the pan. During the 6-7 minute grilling session at 450 degrees fahrenheit, flip the chicken halfway (232 degrees celsius).
3. While the chicken cooks, place bowls of tomato sauce and spice mix on the table. When the chicken is finished, remove it from the pan and discard the cooking liquid.
4. In a small saucepan over low heat, melt the butter. Jalapeno and garlic need to be sautéed until fragrant. When the stew starts to smell good, add the spice mix and simmer for a further 1-2 minutes, stirring periodically. Once the jalapeño has been taken out, throw it away.
5. Add the tomato sauce and thoroughly combine. Salt to taste, then boil for an additional two minutes to thicken the sauce. Remove the chicken from the fire and mix it into the sauce after it has finished cooking.

6. Before using the oven, it is advised that it be heated to 450 degrees fahrenheit (232 degrees celsius). Pizza dough should be placed on a pizza pan that has been lightly greased with olive oil. Sauce or gravy should be applied to the pizza dough. Add a quarter cup of cheese on top. Place the chicken and pizza together. Add some chopped cilantro, thinly sliced onions, and any remaining cheese to finish it off.

7. Lower the oven's temperature to 425 degrees fahrenheit (218 degrees celsius). Bake the pizza for 8 to 10 minutes on the oven's timer. Take the pizza out of the oven once it has finished cooking, then top it with the remaining cilantro that has been chopped.

One pan balsamic chicken and veggies

Prep time: 10 minutes
Cook time: 20 minutes

Ingredients

- 6 tbsp balsamic vinegar
- 1/2 cup of zesty italian dressing
- 1.25 pounds of chicken tenders
- 2 heads broccoli
- 1 cup of baby carrots
- 1/2 pint cherry tomatoes
- 1 tsp italian seasoning
- 3 tbsp olive oil
- 1/2 tsp garlic powder
- Optional: fresh parsley, salt, and pepper

Instructions

1. Preheat the oven to 400°f. Prepare a large baking sheet by spraying it with nonstick spray (or coating it with parchment paper if your tray isn't already nonstick) to avoid the balsamic and italian spice mixture from sticking.

2. Combine the spicy italian dressing and balsamic vinegar in a blender.

3. Trim the tenderloins of any excess fat and gristle. Alternately, cut the breasts into quarter- to half-inch-thick, bite-sized chunks.

4. Place the chicken tenders in a big plastic bag along with 1/3 cup of the italian spice and balsamic vinegar mixture, and shake vigorously. Marinate for a minimum of 30 minutes and a maximum of 6 hours, coating and chilling in between.

5. Separate the broccoli into bite-sized pieces. Cut the little carrots in half lengthwise.

6. Arrange broccoli, carrots, and cherry tomatoes on the baking sheet that has been prepped (would you want your tomatoes to be less roasted? After the broccoli and carrots have cooked for 5 to 10 minutes, toss in. They are already pretty soft, unless specifically specified differently.) Garlic powder, olive oil, italian seasoning, and more salt and pepper to taste.

7. The veggies just need to cook for ten to fifteen minutes.

8. Remove it from the oven, then turn it over. As seen in the video, arrange the veggies on the tray's two sides, followed by the chicken tenders (just touched by marinade). Use 1/3 cup of the balsamic and italian concoction to coat the chicken.

9. Depending on the size of your chicken, put back in the oven and cook for a further 7 to 15 minutes. You must keep a close eye on the chicken to prevent overcooking. The size of the chicken has a big impact on how long it takes to cook.

10. The remaining chicken and veggies may be served with the balsamic and italian sauce. Before serving, those who would like might garnish with freshly chopped parsley.

11. Excellent with quinoa or rice as a grain.

Turkey avocado roll-ups

prep time: 10 minutes
cook time :1 minute

Ingredients

- 2 large tortillas or wraps
- 1/2 cup of simply avocado dip and spread your choice of flavor
- 1/2 lb thinly sliced smoked turkey
- 1 1/4 cup of spinach leaves
- 4 slices of swiss cheese
- 3 slices bacon

Instructions

1. Lay out the tortillas. Each tortilla should include a quarter cup of simply avocado.
2. Place the turkey, spinach, swiss cheese, and bacon on one-third of the tortilla after spreading half of the avocado on it.
3. After gathering your garnishes, roll the tortilla starting at the end.
4. To serve, slice the dish into pinwheels.

Asian chicken cranberry salad

Prep time: 15 mins
Total time: 15 mins

Ingredients

- 2 small bags of coleslaw mix
- 4 cups of rotisserie chicken, finely chopped
- 1 ½ cup of toasted sliced almonds,
- 1 ½ cup of dried cranberries
- ¾ cup of red onion, finely diced
- 1 cup of sesame sticks
- 1 ½ cup of chopped cilantro

- 1-2 small cans of mandarin oranges, drained
- ¼ cup of black sesame seeds
- 1 cup of extra-virgin olive oil
- ½ cup of balsamic vinegar
- 4 tbsp. Low-sodium soy sauce
- 3-4 cloves garlic, chopped
- 4 tbsp. Honey or brown sugar
- 4 tbsp. Minced ginger
- 2 tsp. Toasted sesame oil

Instructions

1. A large dish is piled with cabbage, chicken, almonds, cashews, cranberries, red onion, sesame seeds, sesame sticks (optional), and fresh cilantro. Mandarin oranges need to be included (optional).

2. Combine the sesame oil, garlic, honey, balsamic vinegar, olive oil, and ginger in a blender. Add 3 tablespoons of water. Blend until completely smooth.

3. Drizzle the dressing sparingly over the ingredients for a more or less sloppy salad. After a quick toss, serve.

Creamy chicken and summer squash

Ingredients

- 4 small chicken breasts, boneless, skinless
- Sea salt and pepper as needed
- 1/4 cup of almond or coconut flour
- 2 garlic cloves, minced
- 1 small yellow onion, sliced
- 1/2 lb. Button mushrooms
- 4 small yellow squash
- 2 tbsp coconut or olive oil
- 1/2 cup of low sodium chicken broth
- 1/2 cup of coconut cream
- 2 cups fresh baby spinach
- Chopped parsley for garnish

Instructions

1. To start, warm 2 tablespoons of oil in a big pan over medium heat.
2. Season the chicken breasts on both sides before dredging them in the almond flour.
3. Get a pan ready and heat it before adding the chicken breasts. Three to four minutes each side are suggested for cooking. Remove the chicken from the skillet and set it aside.
4. You may cook squash, onions, and mushrooms in the same pan with only one teaspoon of oil.
5. Sauté for about 5 minutes to get a golden color. Remove it from the pan and set it aside.
6. Set the heat on the burner to medium. We advise adding cream and broth to the recipe.
7. Bring the sauce to a boil, then reduce the heat to medium.
8. Add a handful of spinach and boil the sauce for three to four minutes. Slicing cooked chicken breasts and adding them to the skillet with the cooked veggies is one option.
9. Combine everything in a bowl, give it a little swirl, cover it, and let it set (away from the heat source) for about five minutes.
10. Sprinkle the dish with freshly cut parsley. Enjoy.

Crockpot cranberry meatballs

Prep time: 5 minutes
Cook time: 2 hours

Ingredients

- 24 oz. Turkey meatballs

- 12 oz. Chili sauce
- 1 recipe cranberry sauce
- 2 green onions, chopped

Instructions

1. In the slow cooker or crock pot, combine the cranberries and spicy sauce. Mix the sauce well before adding the meatballs.

2. Cover and cook the meatballs until they are well cooked and the sauce is hot and bubbling for 1–2 hours on high or 3–5 hours on low. The addition of green onions complements the toothpicks well.

Garlic brown sugar chicken

Prep time: 10 minutes
Cook time: 40 minutes

Ingredient

- 8 bone-in, skin-on chicken thighs
- As required, freshly ground black pepper and kosher salt
- 3 tbsp unsalted butter, divided
- 4 cloves garlic, minced
- 1/4 cup of brown sugar, packed
- 1 tbsp honey
- 1/2 tsp dried oregano
- 1/4 tsp dried thyme
- 1/4 tsp dried basil
- 2 tbsp chopped fresh parsley leaves

Directions:

1. Increase the oven's setting to 400 degrees fahrenheit.
2. Add salt and pepper to the chicken thighs as desired.
3. In an oven-safe pan, melt the butter to make the sauce. Add the chicken after that, skin-side down, and cook for two to three minutes, or until golden brown, on each side.
4. Melt the last tablespoon of butter in the pan. When the garlic starts to smell wonderful, add it and cook for a minute or two, often flipping. Remove it from the heat.
5. Combine oregano, thyme, basil, honey, and brown sugar. Re-add the chicken to the pan.
6. Put the food in the oven and roast it for 24 to 28 minutes, or until an instant-read thermometer reads 175 degrees fahrenheit.
7. Garnish with parsley and serve right away.

Crockpot pizza

Prep time: 10 minutes

cook time: 1 hour 30 minutes

Ingredients

- 1 tube refrigerated pizza dough
- 1.5 c spaghetti sauce
- 2 c mozzarella cheese
- 10 pepperoni

Instructions

1. First, apply nonstick cooking spray liberally inside your slow cooker.
2. Make sure there are no holes in the bottom of the pan when you roll out the cold pizza dough and push it into it. The thicker crust formed as the sides are rolled down will hold the contents in place.
3. Add some sauce, cheese, and garnishes.
4. Leave the slow cooker covered and on low heat for at least one and a half hours to create a golden crust and melted cheese.
5. Take the cover, turn off the heat, and wait a few minutes before attempting to remove it from the crock pot and start slicing it to avoid it from disintegrating.

Amish chicken corn soup

Prep: 15 min.
Cook: 50 min.

Ingredients

- 1 medium onion, chopped
- 2 celery ribs, chopped
- 1 cup of shredded carrots
- 2 pounds boneless skinless chicken breasts, cubed
- 3 chicken bouillon cubes
- 1 tsp salt
- 1/4 tsp pepper
- 12 cups of water
- 2 cups of uncooked egg noodles
- 2 cans (14-3/4 ounces every) of cream-style corn
- 1/4 cup of butter

Directions

1. In a dutch oven, bring the first eight ingredients to a moderate boil. Once the chicken is no longer pink and the vegetables are done, lower the heat, cover the pan, and simmer for 30 minutes.

2. Combine the noodles, corn, and butter. After around 10 minutes of cooking time in a covered pot with intermittent stirring, the noodles will be ready.

Easy slow cooker caribbean jerk chicken

Prep time: 5 mins
Cook time: 6 hrs

Ingredients

- 1 pound boneless skinless chicken breasts
- 0.87 ounces caribbean jerk seasoning
- 3 peppers tricolored, chopped
- 20 ounces of pineapple chunks

Instructions

Chicken breasts should be placed in the slow cooker's bottom. Sprinkle some salt and pepper on the chicken. Please add chopped peppers. Put a whole can of pineapple in the dish.
2. To cook the chicken until it is cooked, cover and simmer on low for 6 to 8 hours or on high for 4 to 5 hours. Reintroduce the chicken to the slow cooker after shredding it. Add everything together, then serve. Enjoy.

Slow cooker caribbean black beans recipe

Prep time: 10 mins
Cook time: 10 hrs

Ingredients

- 1 pound dried black beans
- 2 mangoes, peeled, pitted, and diced, divided use
- 4 garlic cloves, minced
- 1 tsp curry powder
- 1 tsp ground allspice
- 1 tsp paprika
- 1 tsp ground ginger
- 1 tsp tabasco sauce
- 4 cups of vegetable broth
- Salt and pepper

Instructions

1. You should use a slow cooker for the beans.

2. Reserve one-half cup of the diced mango for the very end. The foundation of the soup , tabasco sauce, the remaining mango, garlic, curry powder, allspice, paprika, ginger, and the remaining mango. Mix thoroughly.

3. On low heat, cook the beans, covered, for 8 to 10 hours or until they are soft. The mango will soften and combine with the bean juices after a lengthy period of slow cooking.

4. Just before serving, gently stir in the remaining half cup of mango.

5. If preferred, add more tabasco sauce, salt, and pepper.

Slow cooker kalua pork with cabbage

Prep: 10 mins
Cook: 10 hrs 30 mins

Ingredients

- 2 tbsp kosher salt
- 2 tsp ground black pepper
- ½ tsp ground ginger
- 1 (5 pounds) bone-in pork shoulder roast
- 1 tbsp soy sauce
- 2 tsp worcestershire sauce
- 1 tsp liquid smoke flavoring
- ½ large head cabbage, shredded

Directions

1. After kosher salt, black pepper, and ground ginger have been applied to the pork roast, place it in the slow cooker.

2. Add liquid smoke, soy sauce, and Worcester shire sauce to a bowl and add the pork roast.

3. Ten hours with little heat. After adding the cabbage to the slow cooker with the meat and sauce, simmer for an additional 30 minutes. To serve, shred the meat.

Chicken Ranch Pasta

Ingredients

- 8oz penne pasta
- 4 slices of bacon, diced
- 2 tbsp of light butter
- 1 large chicken breast, boneless & skinless, cut into bite-sized pieces
- 1 tbsp all-purpose flour
- 1/2 pkg dry ranch dressing mix
- 1 1/2 cup of fat-free milk
- 1/2 c fat-free shredded cheddar cheese
- Salt & pepper as needed

- 2 scallions, chopped (optional

Instructions

1. After cooking pasta in boiling water, it should be drained and set aside.
2. In the meanwhile, render the bacon grease in a large pan over medium heat. Let the paper towels drain after wetting them. The extra bacon grease in the pan has to be thrown out.
3. Add pepper and salt to the chicken. Add the chicken to the pan after adding some butter. Remove any pink hues from the meat and lightly brown it to make it soft.
4. Use the flour and ranch dressing mix to coat the chicken, then toss to combine. Pour the milk in and whisk continuously until bubbles appear and the mixture thickens. Then, combine until the cheddar cheese is melted with half of the bacon that was kept.
5. Taste it to see if it needs more spice.
6. Before serving, top each plate of spaghetti with additional bacon. Sprinkle chopped green onions on top before serving (optional)

Weight Watchers Shredded Chicken Tacos
Ingredients

- 1 1oz packet taco seasoning
- 4 boneless skinless chicken breasts, halves
- Cup of fat-free salsa

Instructions

1. Fill the slow cooker's bottom with chicken breasts. Taco seasoning and salsa should be used after seasoning the chicken breasts.
2. After the beef has simmered on low for 6 to 8 hours, shred it with a fork.

Thai Chicken Sheet Pan
Prep time: 50 minutes
Cook time: 20 minutes
Ingredients

- 4-5 boneless skinless chicken breasts thinly sliced
- 1/2 cup of chili sauce thai
- 3 fresh limes, 2 juiced, and 1 wedged
- 1/4 cup of soy sauce
- 2 tbsp peanut butter
- 1 tbsp ginger grated
- 1 tbsp garlic minced
- 2 stemmed and sliced red and orange bell peppers

- 1 cup of broccoli separated into florets
- 2 cups of snow peas
- 1 cup of carrots sliced round
- 1/2 onion diced
- 1 t olive oil
- 1/4 cup of peanuts chopped
- Fresh cilantro

Instructions

1. Preheat the oven to 400°f. A large plastic bag should be used to seal the chicken.
2. Combine the lime juice, ginger, garlic, soy sauce, peanut butter, and sweet thai chili sauce in a bowl. Stirring is used to combine the contents.
3. In a sealable bag, combine the chicken with 3/4 of the sauce.
4. Shake the bag to make sure the chicken is fully immersed. Plan to let the food marinade for at least 30 minutes.
5. Remove the chicken from the bag and place it on a parchment-lined baking sheet.
6. Place the carrots, bell peppers, broccoli, snow peas, and onion in a large bowl.
7. Combine the olive oil and remaining thai peanut sauce. Sprinkle everything with salt & pepper.
8. Arrange the vegetables in a circle around the chicken, followed by the lime wedges.
9. After 20 minutes in the oven, the chicken and vegetables should be done. Sprinkle the peanuts on top after crumbling them.
10. Cilantro is delicious on top. You may offer brown rice or cauliflower rice (for bonus points) (zero points). Enjoy.

Weight watchers crack chicken

Prep time: 5 minutes
Cook time: 12 minutes

Ingredients

- 1 lb frozen chicken breast or thighs
- 4 slices of turkey bacon
- ¼ cup of cheddar cheese
- ¾ cup of cottage cheese low fat
- ¼ cup of greek yogurt fat-free
- 1 tsp garlic salt
- 1 tsp onion powder
- ½ tsp pepper
- ½ tsp parsley
- 1 tsp fresh dill 1/2 tsp dried

Instructions

Instant pot directions:

1. Place the frozen or thawed chicken in the instant pot. Close the pressure valve, then fill the pot with 1 cup of water.

2. Manually applying high pressure and cooking for 12 minutes. When you're through, let the pressure to release naturally. The chicken won't dry out as a result.

3. Turkey bacon may be roasted in the oven with the chicken by following the directions on the box. After cubing, store it and save it for later use.

4. Combine the cottage cheese, yogurt, parsley, dill, onion powder, garlic salt, and pepper in a blender. To create a ranch-style dressing, thoroughly blend the ingredients. Until required, store in a secure location.

5. Shredded chicken has to be drained. Turkey bacon and cheddar cheese should be added after coating the chicken with the combined dressing. Combine all the ingredients. You may use the instant pot's sauté setting to assist the cheese melt if the chicken has cooled.

Slow cooker directions:

1. Add 1 cup of water or low-sodium chicken broth to the crock cooker. The chicken will need to be cooked over high heat for 4 hours.

2. Bake the bacon at the same time as the chicken in the oven. Cut it into cubes after it has finished cooking.

3. Combine the cottage cheese, greek yogurt, garlic salt, onion powder, pepper, parsley, and dill in a food processor.

4. Combine the sauce and the chicken shreds. Add some cheddar cheese and turkey bacon. If necessary, you may use the slow cooker to keep the dish warm.

Stovetop directions:

1. Broil or bake the chicken before serving. Boiling it is one of my favorite preparation techniques.

2. At 400 degrees, bacon cooks in around 15 minutes. Cut it into cubes after it is finished.

3. Using two forks or a mixer, shred the cooked chicken.

4. Combine the cottage cheese, greek yogurt, garlic salt, onion powder, pepper, parsley, and dill in a food processor.

5. Use the sauce to marinate the chicken before serving. Add the bacon and melted cheddar together.

Thai Chicken Wrap
Ingredients

Peanut sauce:
- 4 tbsp. Peanut butter
- 2 tbsp. Water
- Juice of one lime
- 1 tbsp. Rice vinegar

- 1 tbsp. Soy sauce
- ¼ tsp. Minced garlic
- 1 single packet of splenda
- ½ tsp. Red pepper flakes

Thai wrap:
- 1 carrot peeled and shredded
- 2 cups of shredded lettuce chopped
- 2 green onions chopped
- 2 tbsp. Cilantro chopped
- ½ cup of shredded zucchini
- 4-5 small cherry tomatoes
- 2 chicken breasts skinless
- Garlic powder, salt and pepper
- 2 la tortilla low carb flour tortillas fajita size

Instructions

1. Increase the oven's setting to 400 degrees fahrenheit.
2. Combine all of the sauce's components in a small bowl. Chicken breasts should be seasoned with salt, pepper, and garlic powder.
3. Combine the chicken and half of the sauce in a plastic bag that can be sealed, then chill for 20 minutes.
4. A ten-minute 400°f bake. To achieve even cooking, flip the chicken over after 10 minutes.
5. Remove the chicken from the oven and let it five minutes to rest. Slice the chicken thinly to create chicken strips.
6. To make wraps, put a tortilla out on a dish or cutting board.
7. Add zucchini, carrots, cilantro, green onions, chicken, and cherry tomatoes to lettuce leaves before sprinkling over sauce. Don't forget to put everything away and enjoy yourself!

Smothered Chicken And Gravy

Prep time: 10 minutes
Cook time: 20 minutes

Ingredients

For the chicken
- 1 pound boneless, skinless chicken breast
- ¾ tsp seasoning salt, or as need
- ½ tsp sweet paprika
- 1/4 tsp fresh ground pepper
- 2 tbsp unsalted butter
- 2 tbsp avocado oil or olive oil

For the gravy

- 1 tbsp unsalted butter
- 1 large yellow onion, thinly sliced
- ⅛ tsp salt
- 4 cloves garlic, minced
- ½ tbsp chopped fresh herbs, use rosemary, thyme
- ¾ cup of low sodium chicken broth
- ¼ cup of heavy cream
- Chopped fresh parsley for garnish

Instructions

1. After being dried with paper towels, chicken breasts should be seasoned with salt, pepper, and paprika.
2. Heat the oil and butter in a large pan over medium heat.
3. Place the chicken in the pan and sear it for 5–7 minutes on each side, or until it is thoroughly cooked and golden brown.
4. When the chicken reaches an internal temperature of 165 degrees fahrenheit, it is done. You need an instant-read thermometer if you're serious about finding out when your meat is done. The thickness of the chicken increases with cooking time. You'll have to cook the chicken in two or more batches if your pan is too small.
5. To keep the cooked chicken warm, put it on a platter and cover it with a dishtowel.
6. Put the pan back on the burner and heat one tablespoon of butter in it.
7. Stir in a sprinkle of salt and the chopped onions. Cook the onions for 10 to 12 minutes, stirring often, or until they are very soft and caramelized.
8. Continue to cook the herbs and garlic for 30 more seconds.
9. Pour chicken stock into the bottom of the pan and scrape any browned bits out with a wooden spoon.
10. After simmering for a full minute, heavy cream is stirred in.
11. Return the chicken to the pan along with any juices.
12. The chicken should be well cooked and the sauce should have thickened after 2 or 3 minutes of simmering over medium heat.
13. A slice of cheese may also be placed on top of each chicken breast at this point, and the chicken should then be cooked until the cheese is melted.
14. Remove the chicken from the pan, top with parsley, and serve with the sauce and onions.

Garlic brown sugar chicken

Prep time: 10 minutes
Cook time: 40 minutes

Ingredient

- 8 bone-in, skin-on chicken thighs
- As required, freshly ground black pepper and kosher salt

- 3 tbsp unsalted butter, divided
- 4 cloves garlic, minced
- 1/4 cup of brown sugar, packed
- 1 tbsp honey
- 1/2 tsp dried oregano
- 1/4 tsp dried thyme
- 1/4 tsp dried basil
- 2 tbsp chopped fresh parsley leaves

Directions:

1. Increase the oven's setting to 400 degrees fahrenheit.
2. Add salt and pepper to the chicken thighs as desired.
3. In an oven-safe pan, melt the butter to make the sauce. Add the chicken after that, skin-side down, and cook for two to three minutes, or until golden brown, on each side.
4. Melt the last tablespoon of butter in the pan. When the garlic starts to smell wonderful, add it and cook for a minute or two, often flipping. Remove it from the heat.
5. Combine oregano, thyme, basil, honey, and brown sugar. Re-add the chicken to the pan.
6. Put the food in the oven and roast it for 24 to 28 minutes, or until an instant-read thermometer reads 175 degrees fahrenheit.
7. Garnish with parsley and serve right away.

Crockpot pizza

Prep time: 10 minutes
cook time: 1 hour 30 minutes

Ingredients

- 1 tube refrigerated pizza dough
- 1.5 c spaghetti sauce
- 2 c mozzarella cheese
- 10 pepperoni

Instructions

1. First, apply nonstick cooking spray liberally inside your slow cooker.
2. Make sure there are no holes in the bottom of the pan when you roll out the cold pizza dough and push it into it. The thicker crust formed as the sides are rolled down will hold the contents in place.
3. Add some sauce, cheese, and garnishes.
4. Leave the slow cooker covered and on low heat for at least one and a half hours to create a golden crust and melted cheese.
5. Take the cover, turn off the heat, and wait a few minutes before attempting to remove it from the crock pot and start slicing it to avoid it from disintegrating.

Amish chicken corn soup

Prep: 15 min.
Cook: 50 min.

Ingredients

- 1 medium onion, chopped
- 2 celery ribs, chopped
- 1 cup of shredded carrots
- 2 pounds boneless skinless chicken breasts, cubed
- 3 chicken bouillon cubes
- 1 tsp salt
- 1/4 tsp pepper
- 12 cups of water
- 2 cups of uncooked egg noodles
- 2 cans (14-3/4 ounces every) of cream-style corn
- 1/4 cup of butter

Directions

1. In a dutch oven, bring the first eight ingredients to a moderate boil. Once the chicken is no longer pink and the vegetables are done, lower the heat, cover the pan, and simmer for 30 minutes.
2. Combine the noodles, corn, and butter. After around 10 minutes of cooking time in a covered pot with intermittent stirring, the noodles will be ready.

Easy slow cooker caribbean jerk chicken

Prep time: 5 mins
Cook time: 6 hrs

Ingredients

- 1 pound boneless skinless chicken breasts
- 0.87 ounces caribbean jerk seasoning
- 3 peppers tricolored, chopped
- 20 ounces of pineapple chunks

Instructions

Chicken breasts should be placed in the slow cooker's bottom. Sprinkle some salt and pepper on the chicken. Please add chopped peppers. Put a whole can of pineapple in the dish.

2. To cook the chicken until it is cooked, cover and simmer on low for 6 to 8 hours or on high for 4 to 5 hours. Reintroduce the chicken to the slow cooker after shredding it. Add everything together, then serve. Enjoy.

Slow cooker caribbean black beans recipe

Prep time: 10 mins
Cook time: 10 hrs

Ingredients

- 1 pound dried black beans
- 2 mangoes, peeled, pitted, and diced, divided use
- 4 garlic cloves, minced
- 1 tsp curry powder
- 1 tsp ground allspice
- 1 tsp paprika
- 1 tsp ground ginger
- 1 tsp tabasco sauce
- 4 cups of vegetable broth
- Salt and pepper

Instructions

1. You should use a slow cooker for the beans.
2. Reserve one-half cup of the diced mango for the very end. The foundation of the soup , tabasco sauce, the remaining mango, garlic, curry powder, allspice, paprika, ginger, and the remaining mango. Mix thoroughly.
3. On low heat, cook the beans, covered, for 8 to 10 hours or until they are soft. The mango will soften and combine with the bean juices after a lengthy period of slow cooking.
4. Just before serving, gently stir in the remaining half cup of mango.
5. If preferred, add more tabasco sauce, salt, and pepper.

Slow Cooker Kalua Pork With Cabbage

Prep: 10 mins
Cook: 10 hrs 30 mins

Ingredients

- 2 tbsp kosher salt
- 2 tsp ground black pepper
- ½ tsp ground ginger
- 1 (5 pounds) bone-in pork shoulder roast
- 1 tbsp soy sauce
- 2 tsp worcestershire sauce

- 1 tsp liquid smoke flavoring
- ½ large head cabbage, shredded

Directions

1. After kosher salt, black pepper, and ground ginger have been applied to the pork roast, place it in the slow cooker.
2. Add liquid smoke, soy sauce, and worcestershire sauce to a bowl and add the pork roast.
3. Ten hours with little heat. After adding the cabbage to the slow cooker with the meat and sauce, simmer for an additional 30 minutes. To serve, shred the meat.

Chicken ranch pasta

Ingredients

- 8oz penne pasta
- 4 slices of bacon, diced
- 2 tbsp of light butter
- 1 large chicken breast, boneless & skinless, cut into bite-sized pieces
- 1 tbsp all-purpose flour
- 1/2 pkg dry ranch dressing mix
- 1 1/2 cup of fat-free milk
- 1/2 c fat-free shredded cheddar cheese
- Salt & pepper as needed
- 2 scallions, chopped (optional

Instructions

1. After cooking pasta in boiling water, it should be drained and set aside.
2. In the meanwhile, render the bacon grease in a large pan over medium heat. Let the paper towels drain after wetting them. The extra bacon grease in the pan has to be thrown out.
3. Add pepper and salt to the chicken. Add the chicken to the pan after adding some butter. Remove any pink hues from the meat and lightly brown it to make it soft.
4. Use the flour and ranch dressing mix to coat the chicken, then toss to combine. Pour the milk in and whisk continuously until bubbles appear and the mixture thickens. Then, combine until the cheddar cheese is melted with half of the bacon that was kept.
5. Taste it to see if it needs more spice.
6. Before serving, top each plate of spaghetti with additional bacon. Sprinkle chopped green onions on top before serving (optional)

Weight watchers shredded chicken tacos

Ingredients

- 1 1oz packet taco seasoning
- 4 boneless skinless chicken breasts, halves
- Cup of fat-free salsa

Instructions

1. Fill the slow cooker's bottom with chicken breasts. Taco seasoning and salsa should be used after seasoning the chicken breasts.
2. After the beef has simmered on low for 6 to 8 hours, shred it with a fork.

Thai Chicken Sheet Pan

Prep time: 50 minutes
Cook time: 20 minutes

Ingredients

- 4-5 boneless skinless chicken breasts thinly sliced
- 1/2 cup of chili sauce thai
- 3 fresh limes, 2 juiced, and 1 wedged
- 1/4 cup of soy sauce
- 2 tbsp peanut butter
- 1 tbsp ginger grated
- 1 tbsp garlic minced
- 2 stemmed and sliced red and orange bell peppers
- 1 cup of broccoli separated into florets
- 2 cups of snow peas
- 1 cup of carrots sliced round
- 1/2 onion diced
- 1 t olive oil
- 1/4 cup of peanuts chopped
- Fresh cilantro

Instructions

1. Preheat the oven to 400°f. A large plastic bag should be used to seal the chicken.
2. Combine the lime juice, ginger, garlic, soy sauce, peanut butter, and sweet thai chili sauce in a bowl. Stirring is used to combine the contents.
3. In a sealable bag, combine the chicken with 3/4 of the sauce.

4. Shake the bag to make sure the chicken is fully immersed. Plan to let the food marinade for at least 30 minutes.

5. Remove the chicken from the bag and place it on a parchment-lined baking sheet.

6. Place the carrots, bell peppers, broccoli, snow peas, and onion in a large bowl.

7. Combine the olive oil and remaining thai peanut sauce. Sprinkle everything with salt & pepper.

8. Arrange the vegetables in a circle around the chicken, followed by the lime wedges.

9. After 20 minutes in the oven, the chicken and vegetables should be done. Sprinkle the peanuts on top after crumbling them.

10. Cilantro is delicious on top. You may offer brown rice or cauliflower rice (for bonus points) (zero points). Enjoy.

Weight watchers crack chicken

Prep time: 5 minutes
Cook time: 12 minutes

Ingredients

- 1 lb frozen chicken breast or thighs
- 4 slices of turkey bacon
- ¼ cup of cheddar cheese
- ¾ cup of cottage cheese low fat
- ¼ cup of greek yogurt fat-free
- 1 tsp garlic salt
- 1 tsp onion powder
- ½ tsp pepper
- ½ tsp parsley
- 1 tsp fresh dill 1/2 tsp dried

Instructions

Instant pot directions:

1. Place the frozen or thawed chicken in the instant pot. Close the pressure valve, then fill the pot with 1 cup of water.

2. Manually applying high pressure and cooking for 12 minutes. When you're through, let the pressure to release naturally. The chicken won't dry out as a result.

3. Turkey bacon may be roasted in the oven with the chicken by following the directions on the box. After cubing, store it and save it for later use.

4. Combine the cottage cheese, yogurt, parsley, dill, onion powder, garlic salt, and pepper in a blender. To create a ranch-style dressing, thoroughly blend the ingredients. Until required, store in a secure location.

5. Shredded chicken has to be drained. Turkey bacon and cheddar cheese should be added after coating the chicken with the combined dressing. Combine all the ingredients. You may use the instant pot's sauté setting to assist the cheese melt if the chicken has cooled.

Slow cooker directions:

1. Add 1 cup of water or low-sodium chicken broth to the crock cooker. The chicken will need to be cooked over high heat for 4 hours.

2. Bake the bacon at the same time as the chicken in the oven. Cut it into cubes after it has finished cooking.

3. Combine the cottage cheese, greek yogurt, garlic salt, onion powder, pepper, parsley, and dill in a food processor.

4. Combine the sauce and the chicken shreds. Add some cheddar cheese and turkey bacon. If necessary, you may use the slow cooker to keep the dish warm.

Stovetop directions:

1. Broil or bake the chicken before serving. Boiling it is one of my favorite preparation techniques.

2. At 400 degrees, bacon cooks in around 15 minutes. Cut it into cubes after it is finished.

3. Using two forks or a mixer, shred the cooked chicken.

4. Combine the cottage cheese, greek yogurt, garlic salt, onion powder, pepper, parsley, and dill in a food processor.

5. Use the sauce to marinate the chicken before serving. Add the bacon and melted cheddar together.

Balsamic chicken

Prep:5 minutes
Cook:20 minutes

Ingredient

- ½ cup of chicken broth
- ⅓ cup of balsamic vinegar
- 2 tbsp white sugar
- 1 tsp dried italian herb seasoning
- 1 clove of garlic, minced
- 4 skinless, boneless chicken breast halves
- 1 tbsp olive oil

Instructions

1. In a bowl, combine the chicken broth, balsamic vinegar, sugar, italian seasoning, and garlic. Whisk to combine. The chicken breasts should be marinated for a total of 20 minutes, 10 on each side.

2. Olive oil should be heated in a large pan over medium heat. Save the marinade juice when removing the chicken from it. It should take around 7 minutes total to sear the chicken on both sides and cook it through without any pink remaining.

3. Pour the marinade into the skillet. The cooking time should be around 5 minutes total, turning the chicken breasts over once or twice. The thickest section of a chicken breast should read at least 165 degrees fahrenheit on an instant-read thermometer.

Baked buffalo chicken taquitos

cook time: 15 minutes
total time: 15 minutes

Ingredients

- 8 oz low-fat cream cheese, softened
- ⅛ cup of buffalo sauce
- 2 cups of cooked and shredded chicken
- 1/4 cup of fat-free cheddar
- 12 6" flour tortillas (my favorite brand is la banderita)

Sauce:

- Fat-free ranch dressing

Instructions

1. Preheat the oven to 425 degrees fahrenheit.
2. In a bowl, combine the cream cheese, cheddar, buffalo sauce, chicken, and chicken.
3. Down the center of a wheat tortilla, spread a line of the mixture (approximately 2 to 3 tbsp). Fold them or roll them.
4. Repeat with the remaining taquitos, spreading them out on a baking sheet that has been lightly greased.
5. Cooking spray the taquitos' tops after placing them on the baking pan.
6. Taquitos should be cooked for 15 to 20 minutes at 425 degrees f.
7. You may dip the taquitos in the ranch dressing or use it as a topping for them.

Bbq chicken skewers with pineapple

Prep time: 15 minutes
Cook time: 10 minutes

Ingredients

- 8 wooden skewers soaked in water
- 1 lb skinless, boneless chicken breast
- 1 medium red onion
- 16 cubes of fresh pineapple
- 1/4 cup of barbecue sauce
- 1 tbsp chopped fresh cilantro
- 1/2 tsp freshly ground black pepper
- Cooking spray

Instructions

1. Soak wooden skewers in water for 30 minutes to be ready for grilling season. The grill should be heated to 400 degrees fahrenheit.
3. Thread pieces of chicken, onion, and pineapple onto separate skewers.
4. In a small bowl, mix the pepper, cilantro, and barbecue sauce.
5. Skewers should be coated with cooking spray before being positioned on aluminum foil or the grill rack. Apply the sauce mixture on the skewers. Every minute, baste the grill for 4 minutes with the sauce mixture. Skewers are turned over and covered with the sauce mixture. After 4 minutes on the grill, the chicken and onion need to be well cooked.

Sheet pan chicken fajitas

Prep time:20 minutes
Cook time:25 minutes

Ingredients:

- 2 tsp chili powder
- 2 tsp ground cumin
- 2 tsp dried oregano
- 1 tsp smoked paprika
- As required, freshly ground black pepper and kosher salt
- 1 1/2 pounds boneless, skinless chicken breasts, cut into thin strips
- 1 red bell pepper, cut into strips
- 1 yellow bell pepper, cut into strips
- 1 orange bell pepper, cut into strips
- 1 red onion, cut into wedges
- 3 cloves garlic, minced
- 3 tbsp olive oil
- 1/4 cup of chopped fresh cilantro leaves
- 2 tbsp freshly squeezed lime juice
- 6 (8-inch) flour or corn tortillas, warmed

Directions

1. Preheat the oven to 425 degrees fahrenheit. Spray nonstick spray or gently oil a baking sheet to prepare it.
2. In a small bowl, combine paprika, cumin, oregano, chili powder, salt, and pepper to taste.
3. Arrange the chicken, peppers, onions, and garlic on the baking sheet in a single layer. Stir to combine before tossing with the olive oil and chili powder mixture.
4. Place everything in the oven and bake for 25 minutes, or until the vegetables are tender and the chicken is thoroughly cooked. Combine with some cilantro and lime juice.

5. Immediately serve with tortillas.

Basil ground beef bowl

Prep time: 10 min
Cook time: 15 min

Ingredients

- 1.33 lb. 95% lean ground beef
- 4 scallions
- 2 garlic cloves, minced
- 1 tbsp. Fresh ginger, minced
- 2 cups of asparagus, chopped
- 2 tbsp. Low sodium soy sauce
- 2 tsp. Asian garlic chili paste
- 1/4 cup of thai basil
- 1 cauliflower
- 1/4 cup of onion
- 1 garlic clove
- 1 tbsp. Coconut oil (or olive oil)

Instructions

1. Cook the cauliflower rice in step 1. The cauliflower head should be cut into florets before being added to a food processor along with the onion and garlic. Pulse food to create tiny grains, such as rice. This may involve many steps, depending on the size of your food processor. To prepare cauliflower rice, sauté it for a few minutes over medium heat in 1 tablespoon of coconut oil. Also effective is a 4-5 minute microwave session.
2. Add the beef to a nonstick pan that has been preheated over medium heat. Brown the meat after cooking it until it is no longer pink, then chop it into bite-sized pieces.
3. Add asparagus, green onions, garlic, and ginger. The delicate asparagus should be cooked for 3–4 minutes at most.
4. Add some basil, soy sauce, and chili paste to the dish to round out the taste. Cut the heat after 30 seconds of boiling. Add extra soy sauce or chili sauce to taste for seasoning.
5. Add thai basil meat to the cauliflower rice.

Beef enchilada casserole

Prep time: 20 minutes
Cook time: 30 minutes

Ingredients

- 1 lb. Lean ground beef
- 1 tbsp taco seasoning

- 2 tsp minced garlic
- 15 oz of black beans drained and rinsed
- 4 ounces diced green chile peppers
- 2½ cup of weight watchers enchilada sauce
- 9 extra thin yellow corn tortillas
- 1 cup of reduced fat shredded mexican style cheese

Instructions

1. In a big pan over medium heat, start browning the ground beef.
2. After the hamburger has finished cooking, combine it with the taco seasoning, black beans, green chilies, garlic, and 1/2 cup of enchilada sauce. Blend after which simmer.
3. Preheat the oven to 350 degrees. A 9 by 13-inch baking dish should be prepared with nonstick spray.
4. Cover the bottom of the skillet with approximately a third of a cup of enchilada sauce.
5. Arrange three and a half corn tortillas on the bottom of the pan in a single layer.
6. Cover the tortillas with the first half of the meat filling.
7. Spread half of the remaining enchilada sauce over the meat mixture. Add the extra three and a half corn tortillas to form a covering.
8. The enchilada sauce and beef combination should be stacked twice. Last but not least, add some cheese shredded on top to complete. Place in the oven and bake for 30 minutes at 350 degrees.
9. Spicy with salsa, mild sour cream, and/or thinly sliced jalapenos.

One pot skillet lasagna

Prep time: 15 minutes
Cook time: 10 minutes

Ingredients

- 1 lb. 96% lean ground beef
- 1 tsp minced dry onions
- 5 oz. Uncooked "no yolk" egg noodles
- 1 cup of water
- 2 cups of sugar added prego italian sauce
- 1/2 cup of fat-free ricotta cheese or part-skim ricotta cheese
- 1 tsp dried parsley
- 2 oz. Light shredded mozzarella cheese
- 2 tbsp grated parmesan cheese

Instructions

1. Use nonstick frying spray to coat a large pan before adding ground beef and diced onion. Until the meat is no longer pink, the steak should be cooked over medium heat. Noodles, water, and marinara should all be well combined.
2. Heat the mixture to a boil over a high heat source. The noodles should be simmered at a low temperature with the cover on for 6 to 8 minutes. A regular stirring
3. You may combine the ricotta, parmesan, and parsley in a small bowl. Add some mozzarella cheese after that.
4. Top the cooked spaghetti with spoonfuls of the cheese mixture. Cook for a few more minutes, or until the cheeses start to melt.
5. Turn the heat off. Enjoy

Roast lamb with garlic

Ingredients

- 1 onion
- 1 carrot
- 1 whole celery
- 350ml dry white wine
- 4 garlic cloves
- 20g flat-leaf parsley
- 50g unsalted butter, softened
- 1 unwaxed lemon, zested
- 1·75kg leg of lamb
- 450ml chicken stock
- 1 tsp caster sugar
- 1 tsp cornflour, optional

Method

1. Set the oven to gas 4, 180 degrees celsius, or fan 160 degrees celsius. The onion, carrot, and celery should all be roughly chopped before being combined with 150 ml of wine in a large roasting pan.
2. Very finely cut the parsley and garlic. Butter should be seasoned as required after adding the minced garlic and lemon zest.
3. Use a sharp knife to make 2.5 cm apart deep incisions in the meat of the lamb's legs after seasoning it. Hand-inject the parsley solution into the wounds. 40 minutes per kg, 20 minutes each lb, plus an additional 20 minutes, should be used to determine how long to roast the lamb and vegetables. The lamb must have a golden brown skin and a pink inside.

4. Take the lamb out of the roasting pan and set it aside. With a spoon, scrape away any fatty buildup from the can before incorporating the remaining wine. Boil the contents of the can in a saucepan until the juices have been reduced by half. Boiling the stock and sugar for ten minutes on low heat. The required thickness of the gravy may be achieved by combining corn flour and a little quantity of water and whisking it into the mixture. Seasoned gravy may be strained into a jug. Serving ideas include roasted vegetables wrapped in sauce and sliced meat.

Slow cooker pulled pork tacos
Ingredients
- 95g jar chipotle chili and smoked paprika paste
- 1 tsp oregano
- 1 tsp garlic salt
- ¼ tsp chili flakes
- 2 tbsp tomato purée
- 2 tbsp cider vinegar
- 1.4kg pork shoulder joint
- 60ml orange juice

To serve
- 1 red onion, thinly sliced
- 1 lime, juiced
- 10 pack mini plain tortilla wraps
- ½ iceberg lettuce, shredded
- 8g coriander, roughly chopped
- 1 red chili, finely sliced

Method

1. In a bowl, combine the chipotle paste, oregano, tomato flakes, cider vinegar, garlic salt, and tomato paste. Ensure that everything is evenly seasoned and blended.
2. Spread the marinade over the meat and give it a thorough massaging. Place the meat in the slow cooker along with the whole marinade. Cover the slow cooker with the orange juice. Cook in a slow cooker for five hours on high.
3. During this time, put the red onion in a another bowl. Add some hot water and cover it for 15 minutes. Drain the onions, then put them back in the bowl. Add salt and lime juice after combining. Everything should be combined in a dish and well mixed before being left aside for 15 minutes to pickle. The color will change to a beautiful shade of pink that will draw attention.
4. When the pork is nearly done cooking, pre-heat the oven to gas 1, 140°c, and 120°c fans. After covering the tortillas in foil, reheat them in the oven for 6 to 8 minutes.
5. Remove any bones from the meat after removing it from the slow cooker. After the meat has finished cooking, trim off any excess fat with a spoon before shredding it with two forks and serving it in the juices.

6. When the tacos are ready to consume and at a comfortable temperature, remove them from the oven. Every taco ought to be topped with a little lettuce, some pulled pork, some coriander, and a dash of red chili powder.

7. Defrosting and freezing instructions

8. Prepare pulled pork as directed on the box for the best results for freezing, then allow it to completely cool before putting it in the freezer. Then, put it in a container that can travel from the refrigerator to the freezer without thawing, seal it, and freeze it for a few weeks. Reheat thoroughly before serving after defrosting in the refrigerator overnight. Once warmed through, reheat in a pan over medium heat while stirring often.

Pork tenderloin marinade

Prep time: 4 hours
Total time: 4 hours

Ingredients

- 1 tbsp minced garlic
- ¾ cup of bbq sauce
- ¼ cup of soy sauce
- 2-lb. Pork tenderloin

Instructions

1. In a medium bowl, combine the soy sauce, bbq sauce, and minced garlic by stirring. Put the pork in a gallon-size bag, a stasher bag, or a baking dish, and cover with the marinade. Carefully smear on a thick covering.

4. After you've taken out as much air as you can, seal the base.

5. Store the marinade in the refrigerator for 4 to 12 hours. Marinate ideally for more than 30 minutes.

Perfect fish tacos

Prep time:20 minutes
Total time:35 minutes

Ingredients

- 3 tbsp. Extra-virgin olive oil
- Juice of 1 lime
- 2 tsp. Chili powder
- 1 tsp. Paprika
- 1/2 tsp. Ground cumin
- 1/2 tsp. Cayenne pepper
- 1 1/2 lb. Cod (or other flaky white fish)
- 1/2 tbsp. Vegetable oil

- Kosher salt
- Freshly ground black pepper
- 8 corn tortillas
- 1 avocado, diced
- Lime wedges, for serving
- Sour cream, for serving

For the corn slaw:
- 1/4 c. Mayonnaise
- Juice of 1 lime
- 2 tbsp. Freshly chopped cilantro
- 1 tbsp. Honey
- 2 c. Shredded purple cabbage
- 1 c. Corn kernels
- 1 jalapeño, minced

Directions

1. In a medium, shallow bowl, whisk together the olive oil, lime juice, paprika, chili powder, cumin, and cayenne to create the dressing.
2. Add the fish and toss it around so the sauce is all over it. 15 minutes should pass after the marinating.
3. Make the slaw while you wait by combining the mayonnaise, lime juice, cilantro, and honey in a large bowl. Add the corn, cabbage, and jalapeno after blending. Add some salt and pepper.
4. A large nonstick pan should be prepared with vegetable oil over medium heat. Remove the fish from the marinade and season each filet with salt and pepper on both sides. Fish should be brought in flesh-side down. To get an opaque center, three to five minutes should be allotted for each side. Before attempting to flake it with a fork, let it five minutes to cool off.
5. Compose your tacos: place baked tortillas on top, then add fish, corn slaw, and avocado. Lime juice mixed with sour cream.

Tofu stir fry
Prep:10 minutes
Cook:15 minutes

Ingredients

- 2 (14-ounce) packages of extra-firm tofu
- 1 tbsp canola oil
- 3 tbsp low-sodium soy sauce
- 3 large garlic cloves
- 1 small bunch of green onions
- 1 tbsp minced fresh ginger

- 1–2 tsp fresh chili paste
- 2 tbsp toasted sesame seeds
- 2 tsp sesame oil

For serving:
- Prepared brown rice
- Cauliflower rice
- Soba or rice noodles
- Quinoa

Instructions

1. The tofu has to be drained. By encasing the tofu in two layers of paper towels and pressing down on it, you may gently pat the tofu dry. Cube the tofu into about 3/4-inch-sized pieces.

2. Canola oil should be warmed in a large nonstick pan or wok over medium heat. When the oil is hot but not smoking, add the tofu; fry for a few minutes while being cautious to avoid being burnt by the splattering oil; and then season with the soy sauce. During the first 8 to 10 minutes of cooking, stir the tofu about once per minute to achieve uniform browning and avoid sticking. There's no need to stir the pot constantly. The secret to getting the tofu brown is giving it plenty of time to sit on one side. Add the remaining two tablespoons of soy sauce, the remaining two-thirds of the green onion, the garlic, ginger, and chili paste. Then boil the spices for another minute, stirring often, until fragrant.

3. Add a few generous handfuls of spinach to the skillet and stir it around so it wilts and you can add more. Add the next batch of spinach after each batch has been added and wilted. Throughout cooking, the first startlingly large quantity will considerably decrease. Add a few sesame seeds and blend. Mix thoroughly after adding the sesame oil. Remove it from the burner or oven. Sprinkled on top are the reserved green onions. Serve hot over brown rice, noodles, or your choice carbohydrate and top with more soy sauce and chili paste or flakes as desired.

Salmon patties
Prep time: 20 minutes
Cook time: 16 minutes

Ingredients

- 1 pound salmon, cooked, skin removed, and flaked into pieces
- 2 tbsp olive oil, divided
- 2 tbsp unsalted butter, divided
- ¾ cup of minced yellow onion
- ¾ cup of minced celery
- ½ cup of minced red bell pepper
- 1 clove of garlic, minced
- 2 tbsp mayonnaise

- 1 tbsp fresh lemon juice
- 2 tsp dijon mustard
- 1 tsp worcestershire sauce
- 1 tsp hot sauce (optional)
- ¼ cup of minced fresh parsley, + more for garnish
- 1 cup of breadcrumbs
- 2 large eggs, beaten
- 1 tsp kosher salt
- ½ tsp black pepper
- Lemon wedges for serving

Instructions

1. In a pan over medium heat, combine the butter and 1 tablespoon of olive oil. The onion, red pepper, and celery should be cooked for about 5 minutes, or until tender. Add some minced garlic and simmer for an additional minute if desired. Put it somewhere cool and let it alone.
2. Combine everything in a large bowl and whisk with a spatula to make sure everything is spread equally, including the onion mixture from the saute pan.
3. Take about a third of a cup of the mixture and make patties out of it using your hands. The patties are baked in the oven before being transferred to a baking sheet covered with parchment paper.
4. In the same pan over medium heat, melt the remaining butter and oil. Relight the stove with the skillet. Cook the patties in batches for approximately 4 minutes on each side to get a golden brown exterior.
5. Garnish with more parsley and lemon wedges before serving hot.

Ginger soy fish
Prep time: 10 minutes
Cook time: 10 minutes

Ingredients

- 12 oz. (340 g) halibut fish fillet
- 1 tbsp corn starch
- 1 2-inch (2 cm-5 cm) piece ginger
- 2 tbsp cooking oil
- 1 tbsp chopped scallions

Sauce:
- 2 tbsp soy sauce
- 2 tbsp water
- 1 tbsp sugar
- 1 tsp sesame oil

- 3 dashes of ground white pepper

Instructions

1. The fish has to be sliced into thick slices that are still bite-sized. It would be beneficial to sprinkle the fish fillet with corn starch.
2. Coat the fish with the corn starch. Apart from the others.
3. Slice the ginger into small strips after peeling and slicing it.
4. In a small dish, mix the ingredients for the sauce. To ensure that the sugar melts and that everything is well included, stir everything.
5. Heat the oil to the right temperature in a wok or high-heat nonstick pan that has been well-seasoned. The ginger should be stir-fried in the hot oil until it becomes a light brown color. They were taken out of the oil and placed in a basin.
6. Fry the fish in the ginger-infused oil until it is evenly light golden in color. To delicately turn the fish, use a spatula, tongs, or even a pair of long frying chopsticks. Fish fillets are delicate and can easily damaged when cooked in a pan.
7. Combine the sauce with the fish before serving. The dish is now ready to be taken out of the oven and served once the sauce starts to boil. On top of the salmon , sprinkling the ginger and onion. Serve immediately with steaming rice as a side dish.

Honey lemon garlic salmon
Prep time: 10 minutes
Cook time: 18 minutes

Ingredients

- 1 pound salmon
- 2 tbsp butter, melted
- 2 tbsp honey (or sub-pure maple syrup)
- 1 tsp dijon mustard, preferably grainy dijon
- ½ lemon, juiced
- Zest from 1 lemon
- ½ tsp garlic powder
- Freshly ground salt and pepper

Instructions

1. Increase the oven's setting to 400 degrees fahrenheit. A large baking sheet may be prepared by lining it with foil or parchment paper and lightly greasing it with olive oil or nonstick cooking spray. Salmon that has been cooked ought to go skin-side down.
2. In a medium bowl, whisk together the melted butter, honey, dijon mustard, lemon juice, lemon zest, garlic powder, salt, and pepper. Apply the marinade liberally to the fish.
3. Bake the salmon for 15 to 20 minutes, or until it flakes easily when tested with a fork, for the best results. 16 to 18 minutes is where i want to be. Enjoy yourself right now.

Conclusion

In conclusion, the Weight Watchers New PersonalPoints Cookbook 2024 Edition is a groundbreaking and comprehensive resource that empowers individuals to achieve their health and wellness goals. With its innovative approach to personalized nutrition, extensive recipe collection, and user-friendly design, this cookbook is set to revolutionize the way people think about healthy eating and weight management.

One of the most remarkable aspects of this cookbook is its focus on personalization. By introducing the concept of PersonalPoints, Weight Watchers has taken a giant leap forward in customizing the dietary experience for every individual. No longer are people constrained by generic meal plans and calorie counts; instead, they can tailor their eating habits to match their unique needs and preferences. This level of personalization not only enhances the effectiveness of the program but also promotes a sense of empowerment and ownership over one's health journey.

The cookbook's rich collection of recipes is a testament to its commitment to providing delicious and nutritious meal options. From hearty breakfasts to indulgent desserts, every dish has been carefully crafted to balance flavor, texture, and nutritional value. The inclusion of diverse cuisines and dietary preferences ensures that there is something for everyone, making the process of adopting a healthier lifestyle more accessible and enjoyable.

Furthermore, the cookbook goes beyond just providing recipes; it educates readers about the fundamentals of nutrition and portion control. Understanding the nutritional value of different foods and learning how to make mindful choices is essential for long-term success. The educational content in the cookbook equips readers with the knowledge they need to make informed decisions about their diet, fostering a deeper understanding of the relationship between food and health.

The emphasis on holistic wellness is another standout feature of the cookbook. It recognizes that achieving a healthy weight is not just about what you eat but also how you live. The cookbook offers practical tips on mindful eating, physical activity, stress management, and self-care, acknowledging the interconnectedness of these factors in promoting overall well-being. By addressing these aspects comprehensively, Weight Watchers empowers individuals to make sustainable lifestyle changes that extend far beyond the kitchen.

In addition to its content, the cookbook's user-friendly design enhances the overall user experience. Clear instructions, vibrant photographs, and intuitive layout make it easy for readers to navigate through the recipes and educational materials. The inclusion of meal planning guides, grocery shopping tips, and cooking hacks streamlines the cooking process, making it convenient for individuals with busy lifestyles to incorporate healthy meals into their routines.

Looking ahead, the Weight Watchers New PersonalPoints Cookbook 2024 Edition has the potential to transform countless lives. By embracing the principles and practices outlined in this cookbook, individuals can embark on a transformative journey towards improved health, increased energy, and enhanced well-being. Furthermore, the ripple effect of these positive lifestyle changes can extend to families, communities, and society as a whole, fostering a culture of health consciousness and vitality.

In conclusion, the Weight Watchers New PersonalPoints Cookbook 2024 Edition is a beacon of hope for individuals seeking a sustainable and enjoyable approach to healthy living. Its innovative PersonalPoints system, diverse recipe collection, educational content, and holistic wellness approach make it a valuable resource for anyone looking to take charge of their health. By empowering individuals with the knowledge, tools, and inspiration needed to make lasting changes, this cookbook paves the way for a healthier, happier future. As we celebrate the launch of this extraordinary culinary companion, we are reminded that the power to transform lives truly lies within the pages of this remarkable cookbook.

Printed in the USA
CPSIA information can be obtained
at www.ICGtesting.com
LVHW081254130124
768912LV00013B/1306